VACCINES

Edited by **Farhat Afrin, Hassan Hemeg**
and **Hani Ozbak**

Vaccines
http://dx.doi.org/10.5772/65856
Edited by Farhat Afrin, Hassan Hemeg and Hani Ozbak

Contributors

Guido Castelli Gattinara, Elena Belleli, Luciana Nicolosi, Aneta Nitsch-Osuch, Ricardo Rosales, Carlos Rosales, Andrey Dmitrievich Protasov, Mikhail Kostinov, Yuriy Tezikov, Igor Lipatov, Alexander Zhestkov, Natal'Ya Lavrent'Eva, Ming-Kung Yeh, Yuan-Chuan Chen, Hwei-Fang Cheng, Yi-Chen Yang, Ricardo Benitez, Adrian Cortes, Jonathan Coral, Colin McLachlan, Alexander Cherdantsev, Anna Shmitko, Nelly Akhmatova, Aristitsa Kostinova, Darya Paraulova, Valentina Polyschuk, Rosa María Ribas-Aparicio, Juan Arturo Castelán-Vega, Alicia Jiménez-Alberto, Gloria Paulina Monterrubio-López, Gerardo Aparicio-Ozores, Waldely Dias, Isaias Raw, Priscila Cunegundes, Ana Fabíola Prestes, Eliane Pessoa Da Silva

Published by InTech

Janeza Trdine 9, 51000 Rijeka, Croatia

Publishing Process Manager Dajana Pemac
Technical Editor SPi Global
Cover InTech Design team

First published September, 2017
Printed in Croatia
Legal deposit, Croatia: National and University Library in Zagreb

Additional hard copies can be obtained from orders@intechopen.com

Vaccines, Edited by Farhat Afrin, Hassan Hemeg and Hani Ozbak
p. cm.
Print ISBN 978-953-51-3475-6
Online ISBN 978-953-51-3476-3

For EU product safety concerns:
IN TECH d.o.o., Prolaz Marije Krucifikse Kozulić 3, 51000 Rijeka, Croatia,
info@intechopen.com or visit our website at intechopen.com.

Meet the editors

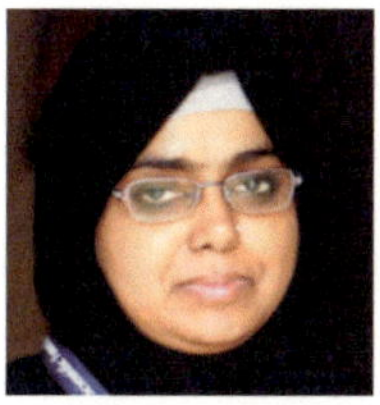

Dr. Farhat Afrin received her PhD degree from the Indian Institute ofChemical Biology, Kolkata, India. Earlier, she served at the Department of Biotechnology,Hamdard University, New Delhi, India, for 16 years. She also workedat the National Institutes of Health, Bethesda, MD, USA, and Centre for Immunologyand Infection, University of York, UK. She is a recipient of several honorsincluding American Association of Immunologists Young Faculty Travel Grant,Commonwealth Academic Staff Fellowship, and Department of BiotechnologyOverseas Associateship. Her research interest is parasite immunology with emphasis on vaccinationand immunotherapeutics of infectious diseases. She has published over 55 papers injournals of international repute and is an academic editor, an editorial board member, and areviewer of several journals and editor of few books.

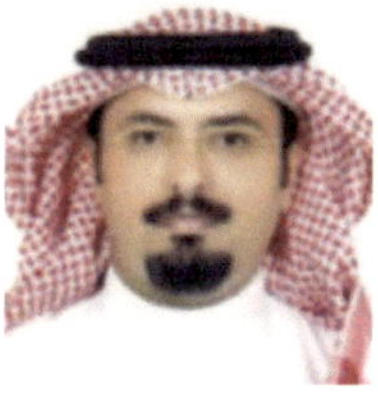

Dr. Hassan A. Hemeg completed his master's degree in PathologicalScience from Sheffield University, UK, and PhD degree from King Abdulaziz University,Jeddah, Saudi Arabia. He earned several honors such as fellow of Instituteof Biomedical Science, UK, and certified Canadian accreditation specialistfor healthcare facilities. He acquired training in microbiology from Sheffield andBristol Universities, UK, and US Department of Labor, Occupational Safety andHealth Administration. His research interest is in the field of antimicrobial resistance.He has published several papers in journals of international repute and is a coeditorof few books. Presently, he is an assistant professor in the Department of Clinical LaboratorySciences, Faculty of Applied Medical Sciences, Taibah University, Medina, Saudi Arabia, wherehe also served as the vice dean.

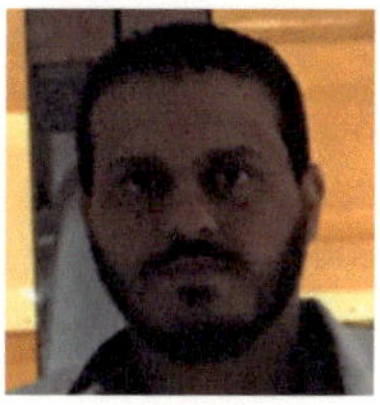

Dr. Hani A. Ozbak pursued Master of Science in Molecular MedicalMicrobiology and PhD degree from the University of Manchester, UK. Earlier,he worked in several government and private organizations and participated inorganizing courses and workshops for Saudi students at the University of Manchester,where he also volunteered as a chairman of Saudi Academics Society. His research interest is in the field of molecular diagnosis of bacterial infections.He has published several papers in journals of international repute and is a coeditorof few books. Currently, he is an assistant professor in the Department of Clinical LaboratorySciences, Faculty of Applied Medical Sciences, Taibah University, Medina, Saudi Arabia, wherehe formerly served as the head of the Department and the vice dean.

Contents

Preface VII

Section 1 Cocoon Immunization Strategy 1

Chapter 1 **Cocoon Strategy of Vaccinations: Benefits and Limitations 3**
Aneta Nitsch-Osuch

Section 2 Prospects for Prophylactic and Therapeutic Vaccines 23

Chapter 2 **Prophylactic and Therapeutic Vaccines against Human Papillomavirus Infections 25**
Carlos Rosales and Ricardo Rosales

Section 3 Adjuvants for Human Vaccines 53

Chapter 3 **Anogenital Warts: New Opportunities for Prevention and Treatment 55**
Andrey Dmitrievich Protasov, Alexander Victorovich Zhestkov, Yuriy Vladimirovich Tezikov, Igor Stanislavovich Lipatov, Mikhail Petrovich Kostinov and Natal'ya Evgenievna Lavrent'eva

Chapter 4 **The Efficacy of Immunoadjuvant-Containing Influenza Vaccines in Pregnancy 67**
Kostinov Mikhail Petrovich, Cherdantsev Alexander Petrovich, Shmitko Anna Dmitrievna, Akhmatova Nelly Kimovna, Kostinova Aristitsa Mikhailovna, Praulova Darya Alexandrovna, Polyschuk Valentina Borisovna, Protasov Andrey Dmitrievich, Zhestkov Alexander Victorovich and Tezikov Yuriy Vladimirovich

Section 4 Biotechnological Approaches to Vaccine Production 95

Chapter 5 **Biotechnologies Applied in Biomedical Vaccines 97**
Yuan-Chuan Chen, Hwei-Fang Cheng, Yi-Chen Yang and Ming-Kung Yeh

Section 5 Engineering Effective Vaccines 111

Chapter 6 **The Use of Planar Electromagnetic Fields in Effective Vaccine Design 113**
Adrián Cortés, Jonathan Coral, Colin McLachlan and Ricardo Benítez

Chapter 7 **The Impact of Bioinformatics on Vaccine Design and Development 123**
Ribas-Aparicio Rosa María, Castelán-Vega Juan Arturo, Jiménez-Alberto Alicia, Monterrubio-López Gloria Paulina and Aparicio-Ozores Gerardo

Section 6 Resolving Pertussis Resurgence 147

Chapter 8 **Immunization against Pertussis: An Almost Solved Problem or a Headache in Public Health 149**
Waldely de Oliveira Dias, Ana Fabíola R.O. Prestes, Priscila S. Cunegundes, Eliane P. Silva and Isaias Raw

Section 7 Vaccine Side Effects 165

Chapter 9 **Adverse Events Related to Vaccination (VAEs): How to Manage the Further Doses of Immunization and Parents' Hesitancy 167**
Guido Castelli Gattinara, Elena Bellelli, Donatella F. Angelone, Veronica Santilli and Luciana Nicolosi

Preface

The human body is under continuous attack by invaders — the disease-causing microorganisms. While most are treated with chemotherapeutic drugs, there are quite a few infectious diseases wherein the causative microbes have developed resistance to the existing antibiotic arsenal. Cure for such diseases is inevitable as it may result in high morbidity and mortality, if not properly treated.

Prevention is better than cure. Vaccination represents the most cost-effective way for disease prevention. Vaccines are composed of components of the microbe that can activate the host immune system. But the witty microbes have evolved strategies to elude the host's defenses. The new-generation vaccines have been designed to activate the immune cells so as to counteract such immune evasiveness. T cells and/or B cells are required to generate effective immune responses. Just like obedient soldiers patrolling the nation to ward off its enemies, these sentinels of the immune system including the macrophages and dendritic cells are activated to release a battery of effector molecules and cytokines, to thwart the infection.

Vaccines are now available against a multitude of diseases. But there has been resurgence of pertussis despite vaccination. The memory response needs to be induced in order to elicit long-lasting protection. The concept of herd immunity or cocooning vaccines is also looming large, an effort to make majority of the population immune to a particular endemic disease. Besides prophylactic (preventive) vaccines, therapeutic vaccines against reemerging infectious diseases have also surfaced.

This book encompasses a broad overview of the traditional and new-generation biotechnological vaccines in clinical use. The use of adjuvants has also been exemplified with reference to pertussis vaccines. The resurgence of pertussis after vaccination leaves us with a thought on the use of whole-cell vaccines for induction of effective immunity. The concept of cocoon vaccination has also been introduced along with the adverse side effects of vaccines. The use of bioinformatic approach for designing vaccines also sheds some information on increasing the effectiveness of currently available vaccines. Further, engineering molecular pattern interactions allow stable coupling of antigenic peptide-MHC to TCR of T cells. Finally, the prospects of therapeutic vaccines have also been discussed in addition to prophylactic vaccines.

Farhat Afrin
Assistant Professor
Department of Clinical Laboratory Sciences
Faculty of Applied Medical Sciences
Taibah University, Medina
Kingdom of Saudi Arabia

Section 1

Cocoon Immunization Strategy

Chapter 1

Cocoon Strategy of Vaccinations: Benefits and Limitations

Aneta Nitsch-Osuch

Additional information is available at the end of the chapter

http://dx.doi.org/10.5772/intechopen.68890

Abstract

A cocoon vaccination strategy refers to vaccinations in persons from the immediate environment of those patients who might develop an illness (they are susceptible to illnesses) but cannot be vaccinated due to permanent or temporary medical contraindications to a vaccination (e.g. immunosuppressed patients) or are too young to have a vaccination. Most frequently, a cocoon vaccination strategy is associated with vaccinations in adults aimed at preventing the spread of an illness in children (e.g. pertussis vaccination or influenza vaccination), but it is worth considering whether this strategy should not be understood also as vaccinations in children with the view of protecting adults and the elderly against illnesses (e.g. influenza or pneumococcal diseases). The aim of the cocoon strategy is to minimize the risk of the transmission of pathogens in the environment of a patient who is susceptible to an infection. A vaccinated patient is not a source of infection any more for a non-vaccinated patient. The chapter presents a history, current implementation of the strategy in different countries, its benefits and limitations.

Keywords: cocoon, vaccination, influenza, pertussis, strategy

1. Introduction

Immunization methods cover [1]:

1. routine vaccinations in children and adolescents under national immunization programs,
2. vaccinations in adults from risk groups (due to clinical recommendations, e.g. chronic diseases, and epidemiological recommendations, e.g. occupation, scheduled travels),

3. ring vaccination strategy (vaccination of a ring of close contacts of an ill person; it is a strategy used to stop an epidemic, as in the case of smallpox eradication in India) and
4. cocoon vaccination strategy.

A cocoon vaccination strategy refers to vaccinations in persons from the immediate environment of those patients who might develop an illness (they are susceptible to illnesses) but cannot be vaccinated due to permanent or temporary medical contraindications to a vaccination (e.g. patients in immunosuppression) or are too young to have a vaccination [1].

Most frequently, a cocoon vaccination strategy is associated with vaccinations in adults aimed at preventing the spread of an illness in children (e.g. pertussis vaccination or influenza vaccination), but it is worth considering whether this strategy should not be understood also as vaccinations in children with the view of protecting adults and the elderly against illnesses (e.g. influenza or pneumococcal diseases) [1].

The aim of the cocoon strategy is to minimize the risk of the transmission of pathogens in the environment of a patient who is susceptible to an infection. A vaccinated patient is not a source of infection any more for a non-vaccinated patient [1, 2].

2. Cocoon strategy and environmental immunity

The concept of a cocoon vaccination strategy is connected with herd immunity and herd immunity threshold [3].

Herd immunity is a term that was coined as a result of observations which showed that the presence of persons immune to a particular infectious disease in a certain population decreases the probability of developing this disease by other persons in this population who are not immune to this disease. The earliest observation of this phenomenon was made in 1840 by an outstanding British hygienist, William Farr, who wrote in his report on births, deaths and marriages in England and in Wales that "smallpox transmission might be interrupted or sometimes stopped thanks to vaccinations which protect a part of the population" [3]. However, the very term "herd immunity" was used by Topley and Wilson for the first time. In their studies into epizootic in mice under laboratory conditions, they concluded that "immunity understood as a characteristic of a herd should be approached scientifically as a separate issue that is closely related to immunity of particular specimens, but at the same time constitutes a different issue in many aspects" [3]. The essence of herd immunity is that the higher the proportion of specimens immune to a disease in a population, the lower the probability of developing the illness by a specimen with no immunity to the disease. Thus, the term can be used with reference to infectious diseases in which some specimens infect the others [3].

Herd immunity threshold is the proportion of persons who need to be immune in order to stop an infectious disease from spreading in a population. For most diseases, it is over 80% [3]. Herd immunity threshold is influenced by the following factors: transplacental immunity, patient's age at the time of vaccination, age-related differences in the frequency of contacts or in infection risks (as the result of the decrease in the frequency of contacts, the real herd immunity threshold is lower than the estimated one), seasonal changes in the frequency of contacts (the period of decreased seasonal infectivity decreases the real herd immunity threshold as compared to the estimated threshold), geographical heterogeneity and social structure (irregularities of risk distribution in various social groups) [3]. Herd immunity threshold for pertussis is high, and it amounts to 92–94%. However, considering the decrease in infectivity with age and the seasonality of the disease the estimates indicate 88% [3].

Population-based vaccine efficacy depends on a high proportion of the vaccinated individuals in a population. A good example may be measles, a highly contagious disease, which has become a re-emerging disease in countries where the proportion of those vaccinated has diminished (e.g. Germany, Great Britain) [4]. Population protection (herd immunity) resulting from breaking the infection transmission with the use of vaccinations has been observed in Australia for vaccinations against rotaviruses (e.g. after the introduction of common vaccinations against rotaviruses, the frequency of hospitalizations due to acute diarrhea decreased) and vaccinations against human papillomavirus (HPV), as well as in Great Britain for vaccinations against *Haemophilus influenzae* type b and the meningococcal group C [5].

3. Cocoon strategy against pertussis

Pertussis is a contagious bacterial disease of the respiratory system caused by gram-negative rod *Bordetella pertussis*. Infection is transmitted through droplets or contact, and the source of infection is an ill person (there are no carriers) [6]. The disease can be developed in people who have not been vaccinated, fully vaccinated, properly vaccinated or who were vaccinated against pertussis a long time ago, as well as those who have already suffered from it because infection-acquired immunity to pertussis lasts only up to 20 years. The incubation period of the disease ranges from 7–14 to 22 days [6]. In total, the illness lasts up to 3 months, which is why it was called a 100-day cough in the Chinese medicine. The most serious pertussis complications occur most frequently in newborns and infants, and they include pneumonia, other bacterial or viral superinfections, segmental atelectasis and replacement emphysema, pertussis encephalopathy, seizures and encephalitis [6]. Mortality rate amounts to 0.1–4% [7–9].

Since mid-1980s, it has been observed that the epidemiological situation of pertussis in developed European countries, North America, Australia and Japan has been deteriorating. This results from the decrease in post-vaccinal immunity, which is not lifelong, but it lasts for 5–10 years. Currently, the highest incidence of pertussis is reported in adolescents and adults, and the representatives of these age groups are the main known source of infection for newborns and young infants who were not vaccinated against pertussis (in most countries, the first vaccination is given in the 6th week of life), were vaccinated with a delay or did not receive the required number of vaccination doses [7, 8]. It was found that the source of *Bordetella pertussis* infection in 30–75% of disease cases in newborns hospitalized for pertussis was persons from newborns' immediate environment (mothers, fathers or older siblings) (**Table 1**) [9–12].

Author	Results (source of pertussis)
Bonmarin et al. [9]	Parents 55%
	Siblings 25%
	Others 17%
Bisgard et al. [10]	Mother 32%
	Father 15%
	Siblings 20%
	Grandparents 8%
	Others 25%
Wendelboe et al. [11]	Adults 48–55%
	Siblings 16–21%
	Others 18–29%
Kowalzik et al. [12]	Mother 63%
	Father 13%
	Siblings 21%
	Others 30%

Table 1. Adults and adolescents as the main source of *Bordetella pertussis* infection in newborns [9–12].

Currently used strategies for pertussis prevention include [13–15] are listed below:

1. vaccinations in infants and small children, TDPw or TDPa vaccines,
2. booster vaccinations in children of pre-school age, TDPa or Tdpa vaccines, and in children of the school age (adolescents), Tdpa vaccine,
3. booster vaccinations in adults (recommended every 10 years), Tdpa vaccine,
4. vaccinations in pregnant women, Tdpa vaccine and
5. cocoon strategy for protective vaccination, Tdpa vaccine.

TDPw vaccines contain a whole cell pertussis component and may be used in infants older than 6 weeks till 36 months of age. However, due to a higher reactogenicity related to TDPw compared to TDPa vaccines [16, 17], the majority of high-income countries implemented TDPa vaccines into the national immunization schedules. On the other hand, it was reported that the duration of the immunity after TDPa vaccines may be shorter than TDPw vaccines [18]. **Table 2** illustrates differences between TDPa and Tdpa vaccines. Tdpa vaccines contain a reduced antigen content, and they are recommended for individuals older than 4 years of age.

In response to the alarming increase in pertussis morbidity in 2001, Global Pertussis Initiative (GPI) consisting of experts from 17 countries was established. In 2005, the organization

Contents of 0.5 ml of vaccine	TDPa	Tdpa
Diphtheria toxoid	>30 IU	>2 IU
Tetanus toxoid	>40 IU	>20 IU
Pertussis antigens:	8.0 μg	2.5 μg
Pertactin	25.0 μg	8.0 μg
Pertussis toxoid	25.0 μg	8.0 μg
Filamentous hemagglutinin		

Table 2. Differences between TDPa and Tdpa vaccines [6].

recommended the increase and extension of the scope of vaccination strategies and the implementation of booster vaccinations against pertussis in adolescents in developed countries. Special attention was drawn to pertussis prevention in newborns and infants who belong to the group, which is subject to the highest risk of severe pertussis. Three vaccination strategies were considered: vaccinations in mothers, vaccinations in newborns and cocoon strategy. On the basis of mathematical modeling, GPI estimated that routine vaccinations in adolescents connected with the cocoon strategy might diminish pertussis morbidity by 50%. These estimates resulted in national and international expert groups' recommendations in 2006 to introduce cocoon strategy in all countries, which have appropriate measures to do this [19].

Cocoon strategy involves administration of Tdpa to persons who have a close contact with newborns and infants (of up to 12 months of age), parents, grandparents, caregivers and older siblings. Optimal time of vaccination is at least 2 weeks before an expected contact with a child [14]. Strategies of vaccinations against pertussis in selected European countries are presented in **Table 3**.

In 2006, the Advisory Committee on Immunization Practices (ACIP) recommended routine Tdpa vaccination in adults who have or are likely to have a close contact with children of up to 12 months of age. In 2011, ACIP decided that this recommendation should be extended and include vaccinations in adults above the age of 65 years, for example, grandparents, nursery and kindergarten employees as well as healthcare facility staff [14]. Currently, cocooning is recommended not only by ACIP but also by American Academy of Pediatrics (AAP) and American Academy of Family Physicians (AAFP) [21].

It is estimated that 605 persons from immediate and distant environments of an infant have to be vaccinated in pertussis epidemiological situation in the USA in order to prevent one disease case, whereas in the case of vaccinations in adolescents, in order to observe the same effect, a four-times bigger group needs to be vaccinated, that is, 2325 persons [14]. This can be explained by the fact that although small children are the source of infection for other population groups in most infection cases (e.g. influenza, pneumococcal infections), in the case of pertussis, an opposite situation can be observed. Common vaccinations in infants and small children have resulted in the transmission of the disease to older age groups and thus household members, parents and adolescents have become the source of infection [6, 14].

Country	Basic vaccination	Booster vaccinations in children and adolescents	Booster vaccinations in adults
Austria	2–4–6 months	12–24 months,	Every 10 years
		13–16 years	
Belgium	2–3–4 months	15 months	Cocoon strategy
		5–7 years, 14–16 years	
Finland	3–5–12 months	4 years,	–
		14–15 years	
France	2–3–4 months	16–18 months, 11–13 years	27–28 years, all healthcare employees (2008)
			Cocoon strategy
Germany	2–3–4 months	5–6 years, 11–15 years	Cocoon strategy
			Healthcare employees (2003)
Italy	3–5–11 months	5–6 years,	–
		11–15 years	
Netherlands	2–3–4 months	11 months	–
		14 years	
Poland	2–4–6 months	18–18 months,	Healthcare employees who have contact with infants (2015);
		6 years, 14 years	Adults > 19 years—every 10 years
			Cocoon strategy (2015)
Switzerland	2–4–6 months	15–24 months	–
		4–7 years (11–15 years, catch up)	
Luxembourg	12 months	5–6 years,	Every 10 years
		15–16 years	

Table 3. Strategies of vaccinations against pertussis in particular European countries [20].

Although cocoon strategy against pertussis is accepted by caregivers of young children, its implementation is at a low level. According to the data of 2008, only 5% of adults who had a close contact with infants were given Tdpa vaccinations [14]. Leboucher et al. [22] showed that the idea of cocooning was accepted by 97% of parents of newborns, which resulted in vaccinations in 69% of mothers and 63% of fathers. In 96% of cases, vaccinations were done under the conditions of ambulatory healthcare (at a family doctor) [22]. Decréquy et al. [23] observed that before the cocooning program was implemented on a chosen maternity ward, only 20% of mothers and 13% of fathers had been vaccinated against pertussis, whereas after the introduction of educational activities, the level of vaccinations increased to 77% in mothers and 57% in fathers. It was indicated that the continuation of vaccinations is necessary, not only at a local but also at a national level [23].

A few reasons that prevent cocoon strategy against pertussis from being commonly implemented and accepted were identified. It was indicated that to improve the cocooning strategy, it is required to combine parental education with free vaccinations in pediatric or maternal settings [14, 22]. However, implementation of the cocoon strategy on maternity and neonatal wards as well as in pediatric centers requires resources from a doctor to undertaking activities, which go beyond their scope of standard duties, not to mention financial issues related to costs and refunds. Furthermore, implementation of this strategy requires substantial financial resources and the increase in the number of healthcare personnel [6].

Currently, data evaluating the effectiveness of a cocoon strategy are limited. Skowronski et al. [24] suggested that cocooning may not be cost-effective in areas where a disease incidence is low. The authors concluded that it would take 1 million parental immunizations to save one infant death, 100,000 parental immunizations to save one infant's intensive care unit admission and 10,000 parental immunizations to prevent one infant's hospitalization [24]. However, Westra et al. from the Netherlands found that maternal immunization or a cocooning program for both parents was cost-effective and even cost-saving [25] as compared to just an infant immunization program. Healy and Baker [26] found that up to 75% of infant pertussis cases are acquired from a household contact, and cocooning could lead to a 70% reduction in pertussis cases in infants of less than 3 months of age.

The concept of "number needed to treat" to estimate the number of adults that would need to be vaccinated (NNV) to prevent one case of disease, hospitalization and death due to pertussis was used and described by researchers from Ontario (Canada) [2]. After implementation of the cocoon strategy against pertussis, the NNV to prevent one case, hospitalization or death from pertussis was between 500–6400, 12,000–63,000 and 1.1–12.8 million, respectively (after adjusting for under-reporting). Rarer outcomes were associated with higher NNV [2]. The authors also demonstrated that NNV estimates for pertussis vary greatly depending on the frequency of the outcome, including the target age group, the degree of under-reporting believed to be in existence, the assumed vaccine effectiveness (VE) and the estimated proportion of infants infected by the mother and the father. It was concluded that the objectives of implementing a cocoon immunization strategy must be carefully considered if the strategy should be evaluated properly. If the objective of the program is to prevent pertussis in the population in general, a universal strategy should be considered. However, if the objective is to prevent deaths due to pertussis, a large number of adults need to be vaccinated [2]. A similar conclusion was presented by Italian authors [27].

The cocoon strategy against pertussis was implemented in the USA in 2006. Data from two small studies reported conflicting results. One study documented a 50% decline in the incidence of pertussis in hospitals with a post-partum Tdap vaccination policy in 2006 (n = 48), while a 20% increase was observed among hospitals that did not have such a policy (n = 145) [28]. In contrast, Castagnini et al. [29] found no difference in the rates of illness, length of hospitalization or mortality in infants under 6 months of age when post-partum women were vaccinated prior to discharge. The authors recommended that all household members and key contacts of newborns should be immunized instead. There is also evidence that immunization coverage of high-risk groups increases when vaccination programs are universal rather than targeted [30, 31].

4. Vaccinations against influenza in cocoon strategy

Influenza is a severe infectious disease caused by *Orthomyxoviridae* viruses. Influenza in child population is an undervalued, not to say underestimated, problem. This might result from the fact that disease symptoms are non-specific and the disease diagnostics is quite difficult, although accessible and feasible both on an outpatient and on an inpatient basis [32]. It is estimated that influenza virus infections cause 10–40% of acute febrile respiratory tract infections in children annually; however, in closed environments this rate might amount even to 50% [33].

In the course of establishing worldwide influenza in children at the age of below 5 years in 2008, Nair et al. [34] estimated, on the basis of an analysis of 43 studies, that in that year there were 90-million influenza cases in the mentioned age group globally. A 13% of cases developed acute lower respiratory insufficiency (ALRI) and 28,000–111,500 cases resulted in death [34].

Occurrence of severe seasonal influenza cases in children and adolescents is described by the number of deaths and the number of hospitalizations in intensive care units. The actual occurrence of influenza in children is underestimated due to the fact that children who suffer from mild influenza are not even consulted on an outpatient basis [32, 33].

In comparison with adults, children who suffer from influenza, especially infants below the age of 1 year, require a higher number of consultations on an outpatient basis [35]. According to the study, 24% of all outpatient influenza-related visits concerned children [36]. A big number of outpatient visits related to influenza and its complications generates not only direct costs but also indirect costs that are, for example, connected with the child caregivers' absence from work and the loss of earnings [36]. Furthermore, these visits constitute an organizational challenge for medical facilities. The number of hospitalizations related to influenza and its complications in children in the USA is estimated to amount to 0.9/1000 children, and most of them concern children at the age of below 1 year [37]. The risk of influenza-related hospitalizations in children of pre-school age is comparable to the risk that is observed in the group of the elderly above the age of 65 years [37]. The number of hospitalizations for influenza in children at the age of up to 5 years amounts to 5/10,000 children and in adolescents, 1/10,000 persons [37]. A study by Rhim et al. [38] demonstrated that 7.3% of children who reported to admission rooms in pediatric hospitals due to influenza-like symptoms required hospitalization, whereas a study by Irving et al. [39] showed that 5% of outpatients diagnosed with influenza required hospitalizations.

Influenza mortality in children is estimated at <1/100,000 patient-treatment years and unfortunately most deaths (even up to 50%) occur in children with no additional disease burden [40]. Deaths due to influenza in children are rare. In the USA in 2003/2004, mortality in this group of patients amounted to 2.1/1,000,000 [40]. In the twentieth and twenty-first centuries, influenza can be effectively prevented with vaccinations. It is worth noticing that influenza deaths in children occur also in those children who suffer from no additional burdening diseases that could classify them as patients who are subject to the risk of the severe course of the disease. For example, in 2003/2004 in Great Britain, 17 deaths due to influenza in children and adolescents aged below 18 years were observed and they all occurred in patients who were initially healthy [41]. Furthermore, sudden deaths in children caused by influenza B virus infections were reported. The causes of deaths were determined only in an autopsy (concerning intravital diagnosis, there were no symptoms from the respiratory system but from the digestive system) [42].

Cocoon strategy in influenza prophylaxis was created on the basis of data concerning cocoon strategy in pertussis prevention. Justification of cocoon strategy for influenza is different than for pertussis because no influenza vaccination can be used in infants aged below 6 months due to low immunogenicity in this age group. As mentioned above, the risk of hospitalization in infants due to influenza is particularly high, and the greatest risk concerns children aged below 6 months. The frequency of influenza hospitalizations in healthy infants is similar to the frequency of hospitalizations in adults who are in a high-risk group. Therefore, effective solutions are necessary to provide appropriate protection for this particularly susceptible population group. Influenza prophylaxis includes hand hygiene, avoiding contact with the ill and vaccinations in persons who have a close contact with the ill.

In the first year of their lives, newborns whose mothers were not vaccinated against influenza either have no immunity to influenza viruses or they have low adaptive immunity. Therefore, it is recommended to vaccinate household members and caregivers of infants at the age below 6 months. Such vaccinations should result in the increase in children protection through creating a protective cocoon. Not all adults are aware of the importance of influenza vaccinations in adults and in children. In order to increase the number of vaccinated persons, it is necessary to provide educational activities and develop initiatives addressed not only at the employees of healthcare facilities but also at patients.

Time is another factor that limits the implementation of cocoon strategy in influenza prophylaxis. The strategy can be effective only when all persons from the immediate environment of a newborn, as well as newborn's relatives and caregivers, are vaccinated at least 4 weeks before the child is born because an immunologic response to a vaccination requires time. Gynecologists and obstetricians should propose vaccinations to women on their visits to health centers before they become pregnant or during the pregnancy. After persons from the immediate environment have been vaccinated, another method of infants' protection against influenza is vaccinations in pregnant women. A recent study conducted in Bangladesh, which evaluated vaccinations against influenza in pregnant women, showed that the number of laboratory-confirmed influenza cases in infants of vaccinated mothers decreased by 63% [43].

Cocoon strategy encourages education of patients and employees of healthcare facilities. Educational activities might increase the percentage of the vaccinated population. In families, the main sources of infections for newborns and infants are parents and siblings.

Studies show that providing parents of newborns with information on the benefits of influenza vaccinations, as well as providing free-of-charge vaccines, positively influences implementation of the cocoon strategy. Walter et al. [44] indicated that after such activities had been implemented in one maternity hospital, 54.9% of parents underwent vaccinations (vaccinations were given in maternity units and were free of charge for mothers only). Shah et al. [45] observed even higher indicators (86.9–95% in two consecutive years in parents of newborns in an intensive care unit).

5. Cocoon strategy for vaccinations in contact with immunosuppressed patients

Patients in immunosuppression resulting from anticancer or anti-inflammatory treatment (inflammatory bowel diseases [IBD], rheumatic diseases) might not achieve appropriate level of protection after the vaccination (vaccines that are considered to be safe for this group of patients are inactivated vaccines). This is why minimizing the risk of disease transmission in those patients' environment is of significant importance. In particular, influenza, pertussis and chickenpox vaccinations are recommended [46]. Unfortunately, vaccinations in the contacts of patients in immunosuppression are at a low level, which proves that education in this group is highly necessary. Waszczuk et al. [47] conducted a self-completed survey among patients with inflammatory bowel disease (IBD) and reported that the use of recommended vaccines in family members of patients was insufficient (22–26%). There was a statistically significant association between the non-reimbursed vaccines coverage level and the educational status of patients [47].

6. Cocoon strategy for vaccinations in healthcare professionals

Due to frequent contact with the ill, high infectivity of the diseases and lack of life-long immunity to diseases, healthcare personnel belong to a group which is highly at the risk of becoming infected with Bordetella pertussis or influenza virus.

In the case of pertussis, it is estimated that the risk of developing an illness by healthcare professionals is almost two times higher as compared with the general population. Serological results of one study showed that Bordetella pertussis infection in healthcare professionals subject to five-year observations was 2 times higher in 55%, 3 times higher is 17% and 4 times higher in 4% of the personnel [48]. Pertussis might become a hospital infection and its source might be either a patient or a healthcare personnel. Outbreak of the disease in healthcare professionals threatens patients' health, especially infants' health. Activities to stop the outbreak might be costly and disturb the functioning of a healthcare facility. Ward et al. [49] described a pertussis outbreak in a 600-bed general hospital in Paris with 2100 employees. In November 2000, three pertussis cases in the personnel were observed there. An epidemiological investigation showed that the first case was a 51-year-old woman who infected three coworkers. A local committee for hospital infections decided to conduct screenings in all healthcare employees and patients. Personnel with respiratory symptoms were excluded from work for the first 5 days of antibiotic treatment. Eventually, pertussis was diagnosed in 17 persons, including 15 members of the personnel and 2 patients. The cost of controlling the outbreak, mostly diagnostic tests, treatment and the loss of productivity, amounted to over 46,000 Euro.

Baggett et al. [50] described two pertussis outbreaks in hospitals in King county in the United States of Washington which occurred in 2004:

1. In the first hospital, the source of infection was a 38-year-old doctor who worked on an emergency ward (at that moment when she developed the illness, she was in the 37th week of pregnancy, coughing fits and vomiting after the fits lasted for 37 days, and the doctor associated them with the exacerbation of concurrent bronchial asthma). Epidemiological investigation identified five probable cases, which met the pertussis clinic definition of Centers for Disease Control and Prevention (CDC) at that time, and two cases were confirmed. Disease cases concerned two nurses, a receptionist, a close friend of the infected doctor and the doctor's husband. The woman put 738 persons at risk of infection, including 388 hospital workers, 265 patients and 85 visitors. Among them, 600 persons were examined (80%) and 516 persons were administered antibiotics. Furthermore, one patient who was admitted to the hospital for an emergency appendicitis operation and had contact with the infected doctor in the admission room had a positive polymerase chain reaction (PCR) result without typical clinical symptoms. This resulted in testing 95 persons who had contact with the infected woman (92 persons were given antibiotics) and 29 PCR tests (all results were negative). Hospital pertussis outbreak had significant economic and organizational consequences. The costs included diagnostic tests, antibiotics for all hospital employees with respiratory symptoms who had contact with the persons diagnosed with pertussis and excluding them from work for the first 5 days of treatment and

2. In the other hospital, a 38-year-old physiotherapist working in an intensive care pediatric unit visited a company doctor due to persistent coughing fits which lasted for 22 days. Although the cultivation and testing of the PCR material from nasopharynx were negative and so was the direct immunofluorescence test, an epidemiological investigation was initiated since clinical criteria were fulfilled by the physiotherapist. Pertussis was diagnosed and confirmed in three nurses from the intensive care unit and in one resident doctor who had contact with the ill person. It was estimated that 417 hospital workers, 200 hospital visitors and 120 patients were potentially exposed to the disease. *Bordetella pertussis* infection was confirmed with the PCR method in four members of the hospital personnel. At the expense of the hospital, antibiotics were administered to 343 workers and 70 visitors and patients. Employees with respiratory symptoms were expelled from work for 1 day until obtaining the negative PCR result. The costs of activities connected with controlling the outbreaks exceeded 260,00 US dollars in the first hospital and 120,000 US dollars in the other hospital, and they were connected mostly with the costs of overtime related to expelling persons at risk of pertussis from work and with remuneration for additional work for the hospital infection team.

Calugar et al. [51] focused on cost-effectiveness of pertussis vaccinations in healthcare personnel. They analyzed a pertussis outbreak which occurred in 2003 in a specialist clinic in the USA after a 1-day exposure of healthcare personnel to an infant with a confirmed pertussis diagnosis [51]. Three hundred and seven members of healthcare personnel were at risk and seven of them had symptomatic pertussis. The authors estimated that vaccinations in healthcare professionals would prevent over 46% of pertussis cases, and from the perspective of the hospital, they would decrease the costs of controlling the outbreak. The authors concluded that pertussis might disturb the functioning of the hospital and that personnel vaccinations could decrease the number of infected workers and could enable the hospital to achieve savings. Members of healthcare personnel who are at the highest risk of developing pertussis are persons who work on pediatric wards and in pediatric centers.

According to ACIP recommendations, it is advisable to promote pertussis vaccinations in healthcare personnel and to facilitate access to these vaccinations (e.g. through facilitating vaccinations at the place of work, providing free-of-charge vaccines, etc.). Activities aiming at performing vaccinations in a vast number of workers should also include educational activities concerning the illness and its consequences (for the personnel and patients), and informative activities regarding the vaccines, their safety and effectiveness. It is not recommended to do serological tests for pertussis before the vaccination and after it. Recovering from pertussis is no contraindication for the vaccination [52].

It was estimated that the costs of including healthcare personnel, who have a direct and close contact with patients, in a pertussis vaccination program in the USA could be two times lower in a 10-year perspective than controlling pertussis epidemics in healthcare facilities [52].

On the basis of serological tests, it can be estimated that even 25% of healthcare professionals have contact with influenza viruses on an annual basis [53]. Interestingly, 25% of persons who had direct contact with patients whose serological tests proved past influenza infections did not provide disease symptoms in the interview [54]. This might indicate a possible mild course of the infection or an infection accompanied with very few symptoms. Nonetheless, these persons can still be a source of infection both for patients and for other members of healthcare personnel [54]. Infectious disease epidemics, including influenza outbreaks, in healthcare facilities might bring measurable and significant consequences for the finance, for example costs of controlling and epidemic outbreaks (patient isolation, implementation of antivirus treatment), costs of temporary termination of medical services due to cancellation of admissions, costs of employing special personnel to care about particular patients suffering from influenza, consequences for the hospital image—loss of trust among patients, impediments in patient visits and legal consequences—and compensation claims [48]. Healthcare professionals are exposed to infections through droplets or contact with influenza viruses at the place of work and they might become the source of infection for patients. Most of them belong to a group which is at a high risk of the severe course of disease and influenza complications due to their age and chronic illnesses, for example, respiratory system diseases (bronchial asthma, chronic obstructive pulmonary disease), cardiovascular diseases or metabolic diseases (e.g. diabetes). According to the studies, 75% of doctors admit that they perform their professional duties despite having disease symptoms, which indicate a current respiratory system infection [52, 53]. Influenza complications, hospitalizations and deaths related to influenza or its consequences occur mostly in chronic patients, infants and young children (aged 2–5 years), senior citizens and pregnant women [54]. Vaccinations in healthcare personnel are particularly beneficial for those patients who cannot be given a vaccination, for example patients who are too young (infants at the age 6 months for whom there are no registered vaccines—it needs to be stressed that influenza infections have been observed even in newborns), patients with medical contraindications to vaccinations (e.g. occurrence of a strong anaphylactic reaction after influenza vaccination confirmed allergy to any component of the vaccine), patients who do not respond to vaccination appropriately (e.g. persons aged 85 and more, patients in immunosuppression) and persons who cannot be treated with antiviral medications due to medical contraindications (mostly neuraminidase inhibitors). Thus, influenza vaccinations in healthcare personnel constitute an element of cocoon strategy for protective vaccinations [55]. The results of published studies indicate that influenza vaccinations in healthcare professionals in medical facilities ensure a significant decrease in general mortality and flu-like disease morbidity in patients requiring long-term care [56–58]. Carman et al. [56] showed that achieving 50% level of vaccinations in the personnel of a nursing home for the elderly results in the reduction of mortality among the elderly residents by 40%. Individual benefits for the personnel arising from influenza vaccinations are less documented [56–58]; however, it was observed, for example that the number of days absent from work due to respiratory system infections decreased and so did the risk of influenza virus infections (88–89% on average) [59, 60]. A slight decrease in the number of days absent from work (by approx. 0.5 days) was also obtained in the population of vaccinated healthy persons of working age [59, 60]. Salgado et al. [61] showed that the number of laboratory-confirmed influenza cases and the percentage of hospital respiratory system infections diminished from 42 to 9 and from 32 to 3%, respectively, in a group of influenza-vaccinated medical professionals.

Scientific literature gives examples of influenza epidemics in hospital wards which spread in patients requiring special care. In 1998, an epidemic broke out in a neonatal intensive care unit which resulted in disease cases in 19 out of 54 patients and a death of 1 child. Only 15% of the personnel had been vaccinated and 29 persons admitted to taking care of patients while having symptoms of a respiratory system infection [62]. In the same year, 10 patients developed influenza in a bone marrow unit and 1 person died. In this case, 12% of the personnel had been vaccinated and five personnel members were at work with disease symptoms [63]. Influenza virus outbreaks were also observed in liver transplantation, hematological, neonatal and pediatric units (in the last two units, additional risk factors for influenza virus infections were identified: artificial ventilation system and multiple pregnancy) [64–67]. A group of patients who are particularly at risk of hospital epidemics are residents of facilities, which render care and treatment services for patients with chronic illnesses. During the occurrence of an influenza outbreak in a facility whose residents were at the age of above 65 years, the percentage of infected patients in an epidemic season was very high and it could reach even 60% [68]. The facts that influenza vaccinations in the elderly are not as effective as vaccinations in a younger population (30–40% vs 70–90%), and that influenza epidemics occurred in the populations of the residents of nursing homes, where influenza immunization was very high and reached even 90%, prove that it is necessary to perform vaccinations in healthcare professionals in order to protect the patients [69, 70].

Unfortunately, percentage of medical professionals who are vaccinated against pertussis in developed countries is relatively low. According to the studies, although educational activities result in the increased interest in the vaccinations, only a small group of healthcare personnel are vaccinated despite their initial intentions of undergoing a vaccination. Pertussis education for medical professionals could solve this problem. Tdpa vaccine is safe and effective. Pertussis booster vaccinations for healthcare personnel might be the most effective to diminish the risk of pertussis cases and the occurrence of hospital infections in healthcare facilities.

7. Benefits and drawbacks of the cocoon strategy for protective vaccinations

The main benefit of cocoon strategy is that it decreases the risk of the transmission of an infectious disease in the environment of a patient who might become infected but cannot be vaccinated. A universal adult pertussis program does not only serve to decrease the disease in the overall risk of disease among infants (beyond that which might be achieved with a more focused cocoon strategy) but it also protects adults against the disease.

The main drawback of a cocoon strategy is that it is characterized by a low level of recommendation implementations and a small percentage of vaccinated persons, which impairs the performance of this strategy. It is critical to the success of a universal program to ensure that adequate vaccine coverage is achieved. A comparison of various immunization strategies suggests that the coverage of at least 40% within the adult population is required to achieve herd immunity [2]. In practice, achievement of such high indicators is impossible.

Barriers to receiving vaccines by close contacts include lack of knowledge about the disease and the benefits of vaccination, time and monetary constraints, forgetting about vaccine recommendations if previously received.

Although it is recommended to vaccinate all close contacts under a cocoon strategy, vaccinations are frequently limited to mothers, which also influence negatively the effectiveness of the strategy. Vaccinations should be universal and cover caregivers of all infants instead of being addressed solely to the families of children from risk groups.

To conclude, cocoon strategy for protective vaccinations constitutes a valuable complement to universal vaccination programs. Nonetheless, it should not be the only recommended strategy but it should be an element of a comprehensive strategy for preventing infectious diseases.

Author details

Aneta Nitsch-Osuch

Address all correspondence to: anitsch@wum.edu.pl

Department of Social Medicine and Public Health, Medical University of Warsaw, Poland

References

[1] Healy CM. The cocoon strategy. Texas Medicine. 2008;**104**(8):3

[2] Lim GH, Deeks SL, Crowcroft NS. A cocoon immunisation strategy against pertussis for infants: Does it make sense for Ontario? Euro Surveillance. 2014;**19**(5);1-9: 20688

[3] Zielinski A. The concept of herd immunity applied to the evaluation of vaccination programmes. Przeglad Epidemiologiczny. 1999;**53**(3-4):245-255

[4] Kuri-Morales PA, Guzmán-Morales E, De La Paz-Nicolau E, Salas-Fernández A. Emerging and reemerging diseases. Gaceta Medica de Mexico. 2015;**151**(5):674-680

[5] Thomas SL, Walker JL, Fenty J, Atkins KE, Elliot AJ, Hughes HE, Stowe J, Ladhani S, Andrews NJ. Impact of the national rotavirus vaccination programme on acute gastroenteritis in England and associated costs averted. Vaccine. 2016;**35**(4):680-686

[6] Kuchar E, Karlikowska-Skwarnik M, Han S, Nitsch-Osuch A. Pertussis: History of the disease and current prevention failure. Advances in Experimental Medicine and Biology. 2016;**934**:77-82

[7] von König CH, Halperin S, Riffelmann M, Guiso N. Pertussis of adults and infants. Lancet Infectious Diseases. 2002;**2**(12):744-750

[8] Crowcroft NS, Stein C, Duclos P, Birmingham M. How best to estimate the global burden of pertussis? Lancet Infectious Diseases. 2003;**3**(7):413-418

[9] Bonmarin I, Levy-Bruhl D, Baron S, Guiso N, Njamkepo E, Caro V. Pertussis surveillance in French hospitals: Results from a 10 year period. Euro Surveillance. 2007;**12**(1):34-38

[10] Bisgard KM, Pascual FB, Ehresmann KR, Miller CA, Cianfrini C, Jennings CE, Rebmann CA, Gabel J, Schauer SL, Lett SM. Infant pertussis: Who was the source? Pediatric Infectious Disease Journal. 2004;**23**(11):985-989

[11] Wendelboe AM, Njamkepo E, Bourillon A, D. Floret D, Gaudelus J, Gerber M, Grimprel E, Greenberg D, Halperin S, Liese J, Muñoz-Rivas F, Teyssou R, Guiso M, Van Rie A. Transmission of Bordetella pertussis to young infants. Pediatric Infectious Disease Journal. 2007;**26**(4):293-299

[12] Kowalzik F, Barbosa AP, Fernandes VR, Carvalho PR, Avila-Aguero ML, Goh DY, Goh A, de Miguel JG, Moraga F, Roca J, Campins M, Huang M, Quian J, Riley N, Beck D, Verstraeten T. Prospective multinational study of pertussis infection in hospitalized infants and their household contacts. Pediatric Infectious Disease Journal. 2007;**26**(3):238-242

[13] de Greeff SC, Mooi FR, Westerhof A, Verbakel JM, Peeters MF, Heuvelman CJ, Notermans DW, Elvers LH, Schellekens JF, de Melker HE. Pertussis disease burden in the household: How to protect young infants. Clinical Infectious Diseases. 2010;**50**(10):1339-1345

[14] Centers for Disease Control and Prevention. Updated recommendations for use of tetanus toxoid, reduced diphtheria toxoid, and acellular pertussis vaccine (Tdap) in pregnant women—Advisory Committee on Immunization Practices (ACIP), 2012. Morbidity and Mortality Weekly Report. 2013;**62**(7):131-135

[15] Blain AE, Lewis M, Banerjee E, Kudish K, Liko J, McGuire S, Selvage D, Watt J, Martin SW, Skoff TH. An assessment of the cocooning strategy for preventing infant pertussis-United States, 2011. Clinical Infectious Diseases. 2016;**63**(Suppl 4):S221-S226

[16] Calbo F, Dal-Ré R, Díez-Delgado J, Oña S, Sánchez-Prados F, García-Corbeira P, DTPa/Hi 067 Study Group. Comparative trial to assess the reactogenicity of the diphtheria-tetanus-acellular pertussis (DTPa) vaccine plus Haemophilus influenzae type B (Hib) conjugate vaccine and that of the diphtheria-tetanus-whole cell pertussis (DTPw) vaccine plus Hib conjugate vaccine, administered in single injection. Medicina Clínica (Barc). 2002;**118**(1):1-4

[17] Czajka H, Wysocki J. Hypotonic-hyporesponsive episode (HHE) following vaccination with a combined vaccine against diphtheria, tetanus and pertussis (whole cell vaccine-DTPv). Neurologia i Neurochirurgia Polska. 2004;**38**(1 Suppl 1):S17–S24

[18] Torvaldsen S, Hull BP, McIntyre PB. Using the Australian Childhood Immunisation Register to track the transition from whole-cell to acellular pertussis vaccines. Communicable Diseases Intelligence Quarterly Report. 2002;**26**(4):581-583

[19] Guiso N, Liese J, Plotkin S. The Global Pertussis Initiative: Meeting report from the fourth regional roundtable meeting, France, April 14-15, 2010. Human Vaccine. 2011;**7**(4):481-488

[20] European Center for Disease Control and Prevention (ECDC). Vaccine schedule Available from: http://vaccine-schedule.ecdc.europa.eu/Pages/Scheduler.aspx [Accessed: January 9, 2017]

[21] Guzman-Cottrill JA, Phillipi CA, Dolan SA, Nyquist AC, Win A, Siegel J. Free vaccine programs to cocoon high-risk infants and children against influenza and pertussis. American Journal of Infection Control. 2012;**40**(9)872-876

[22] Leboucher B, Sentilhes L, Abbou F, Henry E, Grimprel E, Descamps P. Impact of postpartum information about pertussis booster to parents in a university maternity hospital. Vaccine. 2012;**30**(37):5472-5481

[23] Decréquy A, de Vienne C, Bellot A, Guillois B, Dreyfus M, Brouard J. Cocooning strategy: Effectiveness of a pertussis vaccination program for parents in the maternity unit of a university hospital. Archives of Pediatrics. 2016;**23**(8):787-791

[24] Skowronski DM, Janjua NZ, Tsafack ER, Quakkki M, Hoang L, De Serres G. The number needed to vaccinate to prevent infant pertussis hospitalization and death though parent cocoon immunization. Clinical Infectious Diseases. 2012;**54**:318-327

[25] Westra TA, de Vries R, Tamminga JJ, Sauboin CJ, Postma MJ. Cost-effectiveness analysis of various pertussis vaccination strategies primarily aimed at protecting infants in the Netherlands. Clinical Therapeutics. 2010;**32**(8):1479-1495

[26] Healy CM, Baker CJ. Infant pertussis: What to do next? Clinical Infectious Diseases. 2012;**54**:328-330

[27] Meregaglia M, Ferrara L, Melegara A, Demicheli V. Parent "cocoon" immunization to prevent pertussis-related hospitalization in infants: The case of Piemonte in Italy. Vaccine. 2013;**31**(8):1135-1137

[28] Winter K, Harriman K, Schechter R, Chang J, Talarico J. Effectiveness of postpartum Tdap vaccination in California hospitals. In: Presented at the Council of State and Territorial Epidemiologists (CSTE) 2010 Annual Conference abstract book; June 2010; Portland, OR, USA

[29] Castagnini LA, Healy CM, Rench MA, Wootton SH, Munoz FM, Baker CJ. Impact of maternal postpartum tetanus and diphtheria toxoids and acellular pertussis immunization on infant pertussis infection. Clinical Infectious Diseases. 2012;**54**(1):78-84

[30] Al-Sukhni W, Avarino P, McArthur MA, McGeer A. Impact of public vaccination programs on adult vaccination rates: Two examples from Ontario, Canada. Vaccine. 2008;**26**(11):1432-1437

[31] Kwong JC, Sambell C, Johansen H, Stukel TA, Manuel DG. The effect of universal influenza immunization on vaccination rates in Ontario. Health Reports. 2006;**17**(2):31-40

[32] Kassianos G, Blank P, Falup-Pecurariu O, Kuchar E, Kyncl J, De Lejarazu RO, Nitsch-Osuch A, van Essen GA. Influenza vaccination: Key facts for general practitioners in Europe-a synthesis by European experts based on national guidelines and best practices in the United Kingdom and the Netherlands. Drugs Context. 2016;**5**:212293

[33] Heikkinen T, Silvennoinen H, Peltola V. Burden of influenza in children in community. Journal of Infectious Diseases. 2004;**190**:1369-1373

[34] Nair H, Brooks WA, Katz M, Roca A, Berkley JA, Madhi SA, Simmerman JM, Gordon A, Sato M, Howie S, Krishnan A, Ope M, Lindblade KA, Carosone-Link P, Lucero M, Ochieng W, Kamimoto L, Dueger E, Bhat N, Vong S, Theodoratou E, Chittaganpitch M, Chimah O, Balmaseda A, Buchy P, Harris E, Evans V, Katayose M, Gaur B, O'Callaghan-Gordo C, Goswami D, Arvelo W, Venter M, Briese T, Tokarz R, Widdowson MA, Mounts AW, Breiman RF, Feikin DR, Klugman KP, Olsen SJ, Gessner BD, Wright PF, Rudan I, Broor S, Simões EA, Campbell H. Global burden of respiratory infections due to seasonal influenza in young children: A systematic review and meta-analysis. Lancet. 2011;**378**(9807):1917-1930

[35] Poehling K, Edwards K, Weinberg G. The under recognized burden of influenza in young children. New England Journal of Medicine. 2006;**355**:31-40

[36] Molinari N, Ortega-Sanches I, Messonier M. The annual impact of seasonal influenza in the US: Measuring disease burden and costs. Vaccine. 2007;**25**:5086-5096

[37] Neuzil K, Mellen B, Wright P. The effect of influenza on hospitalizations, outpatient visits, and courses of antibiotics in children. New England Journal of Medicine. 2000;**342**:225-231

[38] Rhim JW, Lee KY, Youn YS, Jin-Han Kang JH, Chang Kim JC. Epidemiological and clinical characteristics of childhood pandemic 2009 H1N1 virus infection: An observational cohort study. BMC Infectious Diseases. 2011;**11**:225

[39] Irving SA, Patel DC, Kieke BA, Donahue JG, Vandermause MF, Shay DK, Belongia EA. Comparison of clinical features and outcomes of medically attended influenza A and influenza B in a defined population over four seasons: 2004-2005 through 2007-2008. Influenza and Other Respiratory Viruses. 2012;**6**(1):37-43

[40] Bhat N, Wright J, Broder KR, Murray EL, Greenberg ME, Glover MJ, Likos AM, Klimov A, Lindstrom SE, Balish A, Medina M, Wallis TR, Guarner J, PaddockCD, Shieh WJ, Zaki S, Sejvar JJ, Shay DK, Harper SA, Cox NJ, Fukuda K, Uyeki TM, et al. Influenza-associated deaths among children in the United States, 2003-2004. New England Journal of Medicine. 2005;**353**:2559-2567

[41] Johnson B, Wilson L, Ellis J. Fatal cases of influenza A in childhood. PLoS One. 2009;**4**(10):e7671

[42] Landi K, Coleman A. Sudden death in toddlers caused by influenza B infection: A report of two cases and a review of the literature. Journal of Forensic Sciences. 2008;**53**(1):213-215

[43] Zaman K, Roy E, Arifeen SE, Rahman M, Raqib R, Wilson E, Omer SB, Shahid NS, Breiman RF, Steinhoff MC. Effectiveness of maternal influenza immunization in mothers and infants. New England Journal of Medicine. 2008;**359**(15):1555-1564

[44] Walter EB, Allred N, Rowe-West B, Chmielewski K, Kretsinger K, Dolor RJ. Cocooning infants: Tdap immunization for new parents in the pediatric office. Academic Pediatrics. 2009;**9**(5):344-347

[45] Shah S, Caprio M, Mally P, Hendricks-Munoz K. Rationale for the administration of acellular pertussis vaccine to parents of infants in the neonatal intensive care unit. Journal of Perinatology. 2007;**27**(1):1-3

[46] Zbinden D, Manuel O. Influenza vaccination in immunocompromised patients: Efficacy and safety. Immunotherapy. 2014;**6**(2):131-139

[47] Waszczuk K, Waszczuk E, Mulak A, Szenborn L, Paradowski L. A cocoon immunization strategy among patients with inflammatory bowel disease. European Journal of Gastroenterology & Hepatology. 2015;**27**:249-253

[48] Deville JG, Cherry JD, Christenson PD, Pineda E, Leach CT, Kuhls T. Frequency of unrecognized *B. pertussis* infection in adults. Clinical Infectious Diseases. 1995;**21**(3):639-642

[49] Ward A, Caro J, Bassinet L, Housset B, O'Brien JA, Guiso N. Health and economic consequences of an outbreak of pertussis among healthcare workers in a hospital in France. Infection Control and Hospital Epidemiology. 2005;**26**(3):288-292

[50] Baggett HC, Duchin JS, Shelton W, Zerr DM, Heath J, Ortega-Sanchez IR. Two nosocomial pertussis outbreaks and their associated costs—King County, Washington, 2004. Infection Control and Hospital Epidemiology. 2007;**28**(5):537-543

[51] Calugar A, Ortega-Sanchez IR, Tiwari T, Oakes L, Jahre JA, Murphy TV. Nosocomial pertussis: Costs of an outbreak and benefits of vaccinating health care workers. Clinical Infectious Diseases. 2006;**42**(7):981-988

[52] Shefer A, Atkinson W, Friedman C, Kuhar DT, Mootrey G, Bialek SR. Immunization of healthcare personnel. Recommendations of the Advisory Committee on Immunization Practices. Morbidity and Mortality Weekly Report. Recommendations and Reports. 2011;**60**(RR–7):1-45

[53] Weingarten B, Weingarten S, Riedinger M, Miles P, Ault M. Barriers to influenza vaccine acceptance. A survey of physicians and nurses. American Journal of Infection Control. 1989;**17**(4):202-207

[54] Foy HM, Cooney MK, Allan ID, Albrecht JK. Influenza B in households: Virus shedding without symptoms or antibody response. American Journal of Epidemiology. 1987;**126**(3):506-515

[55] Centers for Disease Control and Prevention. Prevention and control of influenza with vaccines. Recommendations of the Advisory Committee on Immunization Practices (ACIP), 2011. Morbidity and Mortality Weekly Report. 2012;**61**(32):613-618

[56] Carman WF, Elder AG, Wallace LA, McAulay K, Walker A, Murray GD. Effects of influenza vaccination of health-care workers on mortality of elderly people in long-term care: A randomized controlled trial. Lancet. 2008;**355**(9198):93-97

[57] Hayward AC, Harling R, Wetten S, Johnson AM, Munro S, Smedley J. Effectiveness of an influenza vaccine program for care home staff to prevent death, morbidity, and health service use among residents: Cluster randomized controlled trial. British Medical Journal. 2006;**333**(7581):1241-1248

[58] Lemaitre M, Meret T, Rothan-Tondeur M, Belmin J, Lejonc JL, Luquel L. Effect of influenza vaccination of nursing home staff on mortality of residents: A cluster-randomized trial. Journal of the American Geriatrics Society. 2009;**57**(9):1580-1586

[59] Nichol KL, Mendelman PM, Mallon KP, Jackson LA, Gorse GJ, Belshe RB. Effectiveness of live, attenuated intranasal influenza virus vaccine in healthy, working adults: A randomized controlled trial. Journal of the American Medical Association. 1999;**282**(2):137-144

[60] Wilde JA, McMillan JA, Serwint J, Butta J, O'Riordan MA, Steinhoff MC. Effectiveness of influenza vaccine in health care professionals: A randomized trial. Journal of the American Medical Association. 1999;**281**(10):908-913

[61] Salgado CD, Farr BM, Hall KK, Hayden FG. Influenza in the acute hospital setting. Lancet Infectious Diseases. 2002;**2**:145-155

[62] Cunney RJ, Bialachowski A, Thornley D, Smaill FM, Pennie RA. An outbreak of influenza A in a neonatal intensive care unit. Infection Control and Hospital Epidemiology. 2000;**21**(7):449-454

[63] Weinstock DM, Eagan J, Malak SA, Rogers M, Wallace H, Kiehn TE. Control of influenza A on a bone marrow transplant unit. Infection Control and Hospital Epidemiology. 2000;**21**(11):730-732

[64] Malavaud S, Malavaud B, Sandres K, Durand D, Marty N, Icart J. Nosocomial outbreak of influenza virus A (H3N2) infection in a solid organ transplant department. Transplantation. 2001;**72**:535-537

[65] Maltezou HC, Drancourt M. Nosocomial influenza in children. Journal of Hospital Infection. 2003;**55**:83-91

[66] Kapila R, Lintz DI, Tecson FT, Ziskin L, Louria DB. A nosocomial outbreak of influenza A. Chest. 1977;**71**:576-579

[67] Sartor C, Zandotti C, Romain F, Jacomo V, Simon S, Atlan-Gepner C. Disruption of services in an internal medicine unit due to a nosocomial influenza outbreak. Infection Control and Hospital Epidemiology. 2002;**23**:615-619

[68] Coles FB, Balzano GJ, Morse DL. An outbreak of influenza A (H3N2) in a well immunized nursing home population. Journal of the American Geriatrics Society. 1989;**40**:589-592

[69] Dorrell L, Hassan I, Marshall S, Chakraverty P, Ong E. Clinical and serological responses to an inactivated influenza vaccine in adults with HIV infection, diabetes, obstructive airways disease, elderly adults and healthy volunteers. International Journal of STD & AIDS. 1997;**8**:776-779

[70] Govaert TM, Thijs CT, Masurel N, Sprenger MJ, Dinant GJ, Knottnerus JA. The efficacy of influenza vaccination in elderly individuals. A randomized double-blind placebo-controlled trial. Journal of the American Medical Association. 1994;**272**:1

Section 2

Prospects for Prophylactic and Therapeutic Vaccines

Chapter 2

Prophylactic and Therapeutic Vaccines against Human Papillomavirus Infections

Carlos Rosales and Ricardo Rosales

Additional information is available at the end of the chapter

http://dx.doi.org/10.5772/intechopen.69548

Abstract

Human papillomaviruses (HPVs) are a large family of double-strand DNA viruses comprising more than 180 types. Infection with HPV is associated with benign and malignant proliferation of skin and mucosae. Low-risk HPVs produce warts, whereas high-risk viruses induce tumors. Because there are no anti-viral drugs for HPV infection, there is a lot of interest in vaccines that can prevent the infection and also in vaccines that can be used to treat established infections and HPV-related tumors. Two prophylactic vaccines have been approved for preventing HPV infection. They seem to be effective when very young people are vaccinated. Unfortunately, many older people are still at risk of infection, mainly in countries where vaccination coverage is not efficient and for those people, novel therapeutic vaccines are being developed. This chapter describes the properties of HPV vaccines used today and the current status of several therapeutic vaccines been developed to treat HPV-induced lesions.

Keywords: human papillomavirus, T cell, cytotoxicity, immunoglobulin, antibody, vaccinia virus

1. Introduction

About 40 years ago, human papillomavirus (HPV) infections were initially reported. This viral infection caused benign warts, which in most cases regressed spontaneously [1]. Since then, several types of HPV have been identified. Some of them have been associated with cervical carcinoma [2]. This form of cancer is very frequent around the world [3] and mostly among women [4].

HPV have selective tropism for cutaneous or mucosal epithelia [5]. More than 200 genotypes of HPV have been identified and classified into high-risk and low-risk groups according to their degree of oncogenic capacity [6]. The two most common low-risk HPV are HPV 6 and HPV 11. They cause most genital warts and recurrent respiratory papillomas [7]. The HVP types, HPV 16 and HPV 18, are responsible for about 60% of all cancer cases [4, 8]. High-risk HPV are involved in other types of cancer, including tumors of anus, vagina, vulva, and penis [9]. In addition, many tongue, trough, and tonsil tumors are also caused by HPV [10–12].

Most sexually active women will be infected by at least one high-risk HPV during their lifetime [13]. Most of these infections will remain asymptomatic and are eliminated by the immune system [14]. However, for a fraction of infected women whose immune system fails to clear the infection, the virus can persist for a long time causing lesions that may further progress into cervical intraepithelial neoplasia (CIN) and even cervical cancer [15, 16]. Early detection of HPV-induced lesions is relevant for preventing the development of cancer. Confirming the presence of HPV DNA in the lesion is the most effective way to diagnose HPV infection [17, 18]. Unfortunately, this type of testing is expensive and difficult to implement in poor parts of the world [19]. Therefore, regular screening of cytological (Pap smear) or colposcopic abnormalities continues to be an effective preventive strategy for cervical cancer [20]. Still, this is not easy to accomplish in many parts of the world, and HPV-induced cancer continues to be a significant global health burden [3, 21].

The fact that most HPV infections are cleared spontaneously shows that the immune system can effectively eliminate virus-infected cells. This provides an opportunity for controlling HPV-induced cancers through immunization and other novel therapies. Vaccines have been successfully used as a preventative measure against many viral infectious diseases, including smallpox, polio, measles, yellow fever, and hepatitis B [22]. Similarly, a couple of prophylactic vaccines have been developed to prevent HPV infections. These vaccines direct the immune system toward the major capsid protein L1 of the HPV particle [23, 24]. Prophylactic vaccines have been effective in preventing vaccinated, healthy patients from acquiring HPV infections. They have also been effective in preventing reinfection by the same HPV type. However, these prophylactic vaccines have not shown any therapeutic effects on established HPV infections or HPV-induced lesions [25, 26]. Despite these advances in prevention of HPV infections, there is still a need for treatments of already existing HPV infections and their associated malignancies. Novel therapeutic approaches take advantage of our knowledge on how the immune system eliminates virus-infected cells through cytotoxic T cells [27]. Based on this, therapeutic vaccines and intralesion immunotherapeutic strategies are been developed. The idea behind them is to activate specific cytotoxic cells toward HPV-infected cells [28, 29]. In this chapter, we describe the current status of the prophylactic vaccines, and discuss the several therapeutic vaccines that are under development for treatment of HPV-induced lesions.

2. Papillomavirus

Papillomavirus belong to the Papovaviridae family of DNA viruses. The genome of these viruses is about 8000 base pairs and comprises eight defined genes (**Figure 1**). Six early genes code for proteins involved in virus replication and two late genes code for proteins that form

http://dx.doi.org/10.5772/intechopen.69548

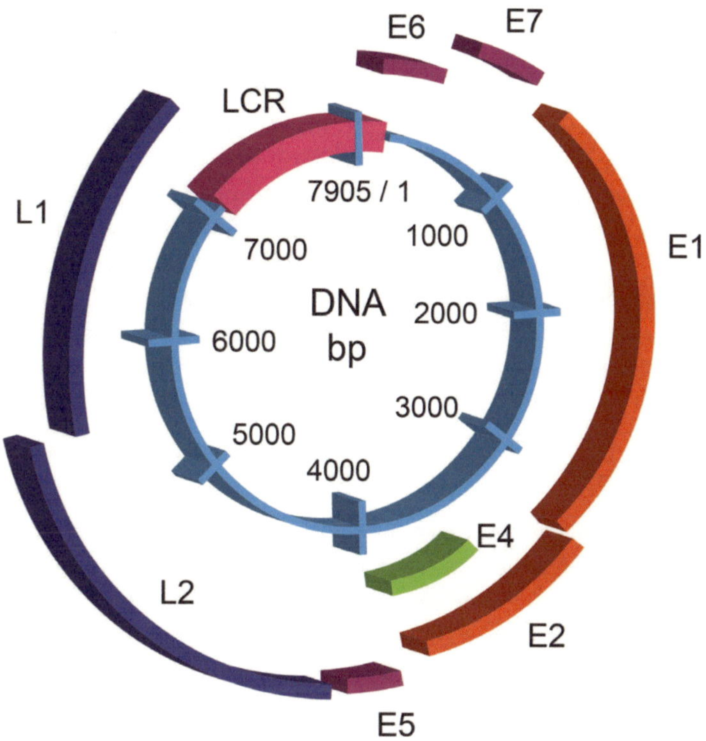

Figure 1. Human papilloma virus genome. The genomic organization of the human papilloma virus 16 is shown. The double strand DNA is about 8000 base pairs. The sequence LCR (long consensus repeat) comprises the promoter and enhancer elements. The early genes E1, E2, E6, and E7 code for proteins involved in viral replication and transcription. The E4 and E5 genes code for proteins involved in immune evasion and virus release. The late genes L1 and L2 code for the virus structural proteins. The E6 and E7 proteins alter the cell replication process and in consequence can function as oncogenes.

the capsid of virus. HPV gene expression is coordinated with the differentiation process of the epithelium. During infection, thousands of new virions are formed and released from the cells without causing cell death [30, 31].

2.1. Low-risk HPV

Infection with HPV is very common and is associated with benign and malignant proliferation of skin and squamous mucosae. Viruses that produce asymptomatic infections or that induce benign growth are classified as low-risk. HPV 6 and HPV 11 are the most common low-risk HPV. Other types are HPV 42, 43, 44, and 45. They produce genital warts and recurrent respiratory papillomas [7]. The standard therapy for low-risk HPV infections is usually the physical removal of the lesion. For this, cryotherapy, application of trichloroacetic acid, laser treatment, or surgical removal is most common.

2.2. High-risk HPV

HPV infections that do not clear spontaneously, usually persist for a long time, and eventually they induce tissue transformation leading to cancer. The viruses associated with tumor formation are classified as high-risk HPV. In this group, we find the HPV types 16, 18, 31, 33, 35, 39, 45, 51, 52, 56, and 58. This group is very important because only about 15 high-risk HPV are responsible for around 95% of all cervical carcinomas [8]. Among these viruses, types HPV 16 and HPV 18 account for about 50 and 14% of all cases of cervical cancer, respectively [4]. High-risk HPV are also involved in other types of cancer, including tumors of the anus, the vagina, vulva, and penis. For these types of tumors, HPV 16 is the most common virus [9]. Also, tumors in tongue, trough [11], and tonsil are also caused by HPV [10]. Similar to most neoplasias, tumor development is a progressive disease. In the case of high-risk HPV infections, malignant lesions display various degrees of histological abnormalities. For the cervix, these lesions are classified as cervical intraepithelial neoplasia (CIN) 1, mild; CIN 2, moderate; and CIN 3, severe. All of these lesions can progress to invasive cancer.

2.3. Life cycle of HPV infection

The human papillomavirus (HPV) infect the epithelium of the cervix, and their replication is closely linked to the differentiation of the epithelium [30, 31] (**Figure 2**). The life cycle of the virus begins when it infects a keratinocyte in the basal layer of the epithelium. The virus usually gets access to the basal membrane through a micro trauma of the epithelium. Once inside the cell, the virus DNA is maintained in the proliferating cells at a low-copy number. During this time, the E1 and E2 genes are expressed and their proteins regulate viral DNA replication and expression of the other early viral genes. E1 is a viral enzyme with ATPase and helicase activity [32, 33]. E2 is a DNA-binding protein involved in activation or repression of different HPV promoters [34, 35]. As the infected cell migrates toward the superficial layers of the squamous epithelium, the viral genome gets integrated into the cellular

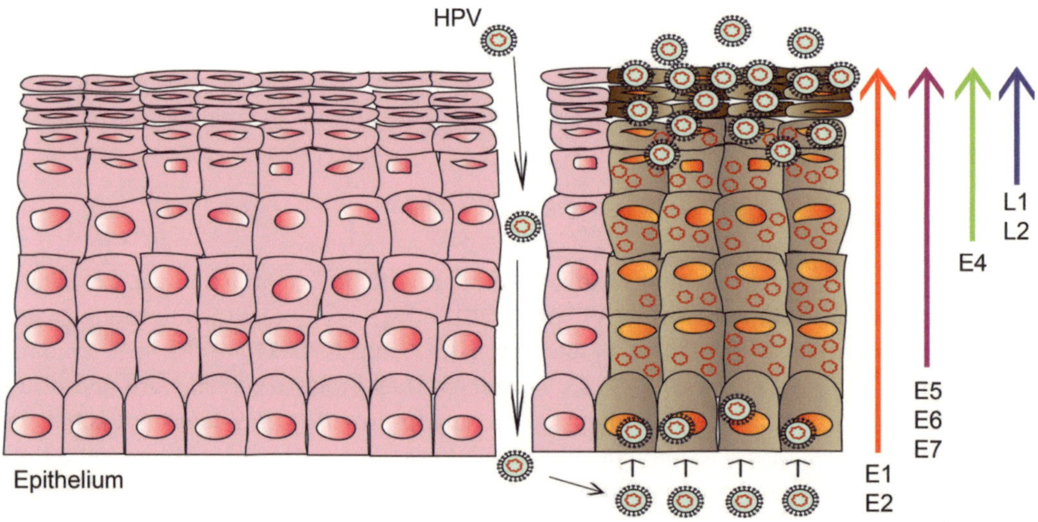

Figure 2. Papilloma virus life cycle. An HPV (human papilloma virus) can reach the base of an epithelium through small cuts and then infect cells. The virus DNA (circles) replicates in the proliferating cells first at a low-copy number, and later when cells differentiate at a high-copy number. In the cells at the top of the epithelium, new virions are formed and released without causing cell death. Expression of the virus proteins is shown at the right.

genome. This integration disrupts or inactivates the E2 gene, leading to a derepression of the E6 and E7 genes. The E6 and E7 gene products modify the cell cycle to maintain the infected keratinocyte in a state, which is advantageous for viral DNA amplification. The E6 protein can associate with and inactivate the p53 tumor suppressor protein. E6 ubiquitinates p53, thus labeling it for proteosomal degradation. The E7 protein binds to the retinoblastoma tumor suppressor gene product pRB, and in this way it competes for binding of pRB to the transcription factor E2F. The result is the release of E2F, which can bind and activate its DNA targets to promote cell cycle progression. With these effects, E6 and E7 are truly oncoproteins and are also responsible for cell transformation [36]. Expression of these oncogenes appears to be a critical step in the maintenance of the transformed stage and progression to invasive carcinoma. The classification of HPV as low- or high-risk types seems to be determined by the relative affinities of E6 and E7 to p53 and pRB, respectively [37]. The E4 gene is an open-reading frame (ORF) within the E2 ORF. This gene product is generated by spliced mRNA and is located centrally within the E2 gene. The E4 is involved in the amplification success and virus synthesis, suggesting a role in virus release and/or transmission [38]. The E5 gene is the least studied so far. Its function is not well characterized. However, HPV infection and transformation take place in complex regulatory patterns of gene expression, in which E5 gene is involved. E5 proteins are thought to act by modulating the activity of cellular proteins [39].

As the infected keratinocytes differentiate and move to the suprabasal and granular epithelial layers, the late genes L1 and L2 are expressed. The proteins L1 and L2 are the major and minor capsid proteins, respectively, and encapsidate the newly synthesized viral DNA (**Figure 2**). L1 can assemble spontaneously into a 72-pentamer icosahedral structure that closely resembles new virions [40]. These pentamers together with the L2 protein form the complete viral capsid [41]. This new capsid gains stability by disulfide bonds between L1 and L2 proteins, and provides resistance to environmental insults when the virus is shed from the epithelium [42], completing the HPV lifecycle (**Figure 2**).

3. Therapy for HPV infections

HPV infection of the anogenital area produces two types of lesions: warts (condyloma acuminata) and squamous intraepithelial lesions. These intraepithelial lesions can progress to neoplasia when a high-risk HPV is involved. Treatment for cervical intraepithelial neoplasia (CIN) usually contemplates elimination of the damaged HPV-infected tissue, leaving the healthy tissue of the cervix intact [43]. Ablative therapies commonly used include cryotherapy, excision procedures (conization), and electrosurgery [44, 45].

4. Immune response to HPV

Protection against viral infections is provided by both arms of the immune system. First, HPV infects cells in a damaged epithelium. The initial inflammation response attracts immune cells to the tissue, mainly neutrophils, followed by macrophages and later lymphocytes. These innate immune cells can detect nonspecific viral molecules, such as double-stranded viral DNA. In response, cells produce inflammatory cytokines, such as interleukin (IL)-1β, IL-6, IL-8, IL-12, and α-, β-, and γ-interferon (IFN), which in turn activate natural killer (NK) cells [46]. Later, when the new viral proteins are produced, these proteins can be taken up by antigen-presenting cells (APCs), such as Langerhans cells or dendritic cells (DCs) [47]. These APCs process the proteins into small peptides and present them together with major histocompatibility complex (MHC) molecules on the cell membrane, to lymphocytes (T cells) for initiation of an adaptive immune response (**Figure 3**). Activated CD4+ helper T cells can differentiate into Th1, Th2, or Treg/Th3 phenotypes depending on the cytokines they produce. CD4+ helper T cells then, on one hand help activating B cells for the production of specific anti-virus antibodies. On the other hand, they help CD8+ T cells to differentiate into cytotoxic T lymphocytes (CTL) which secrete the proteolytic enzymes, granzyme, and perforin [48]. CTLs are the most efficient cells for destroying HPV-infected cells (**Figure 4**).

An adaptive immune response against the virus is important and for the most cases effective for controlling HPV infections [27]. This is supported by the fact that most HPV-related lesions are cleared spontaneously by immune-competent individuals [14, 30]. Also, in HPV-related regressing, but not in persistent lesions, infiltration of cytotoxic T cells has been detected [49]. Moreover, in immunosuppressed individuals, such as organ transplant recipients [50] or

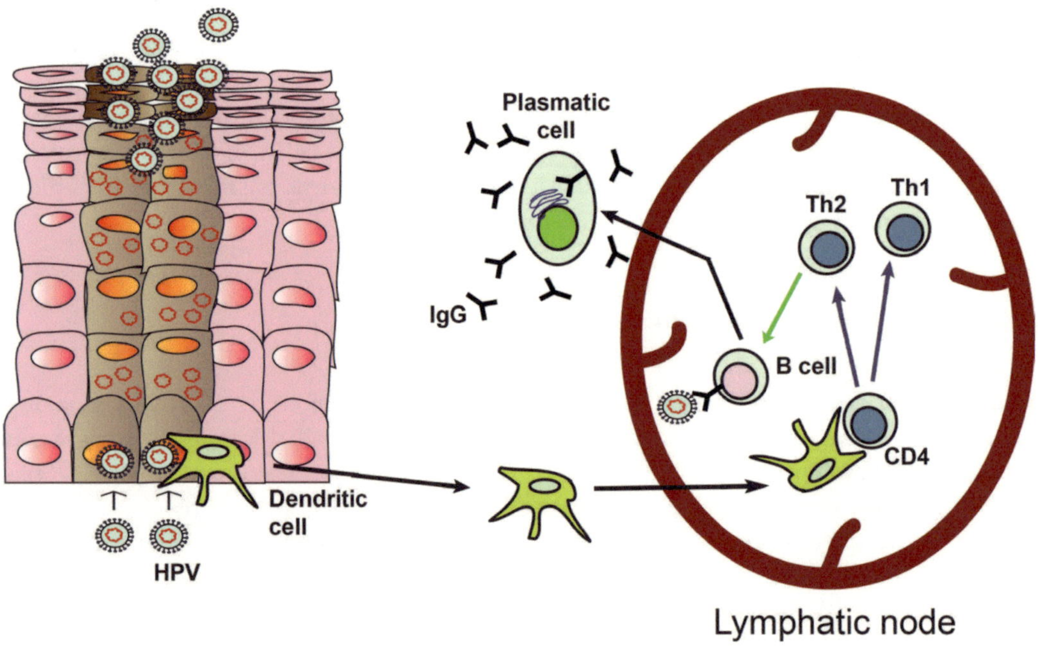

Figure 3. Humoral immune response to HPV. Dendritic cells (DC) capture HPV antigens from infected cells and migrate to lymph nodes, where they present the processed antigen to CD4+ T cells. These T cells then differentiate into T helper cells, either Th1 or Th2, depending on the type of cytokines they produce. B cells recognize native viral antigens and with help from Th2 cells, differentiate into antibody (IgG)-secreting plasma cells.

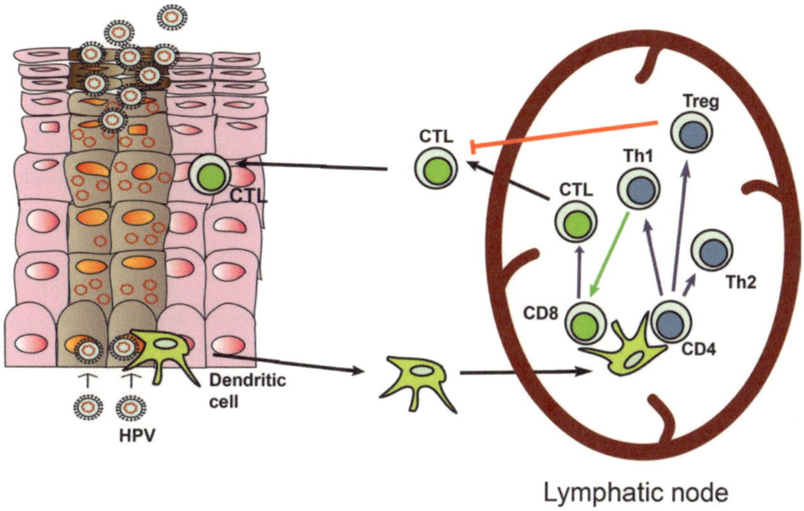

Figure 4. Cellular immune response to HPV. Dendritic cells (DC) take HPV antigens and migrate to lymph nodes. There, DC present processed viral antigens to CD8+ T cells in the context of MHC class I molecules and to CD4+ T cells in the context of MHC class II molecules. CD4+ T cells differentiate into T helper (Th1 or Th2) cells. With the help from Th1 cells, CD8+ T cells differentiate into cytotoxic T cells (CTL). These CTL migrate back to kill virus-infected epithelial cells. CD4+ T cells can also differentiate into regulatory T cells (Treg), which inhibit the cytotoxic activity of CTL.

human immunodeficiency virus (HIV)-infected people present a higher incidence of HPV-related lesions [51].

4.1. Humoral response

An efficient humoral immune response is detected in most patients with HPV infections. These patients have antibodies that recognize viral proteins, such as L1, E2, and E4 the first stage of infection. Later, when the virus DNA gets integrated into the cell genome, antibodies specific for the E6 and E7 proteins can be found in some lesions. Unfortunately, this antibody response is weak and variable and it does not seem to protect from future re-infections [52]. Thus, humoral responses are not efficient at eliminating established HPV lesions.

4.2. Cellular response

A cellular immune response is more important for eliminating HPV-related lesions. Activated CD8+ cytotoxic T cells, can efficiently destroy virus-infected cells, and in doing so they also prevent the onset of cancer lesions (**Figure 4**). The central role of T cells for controlling HPV infections is supported by many clinical observations where the elimination of lesions correlates with T cell functions. For example, patients who successfully eliminated previous HPV 16 infections present memory T cell responses to viral proteins [53], and in patients with spontaneous regression of grade 3 vulvar intraepithelial neoplasia strong CD4+ and CD8+ T cell responses are found [49]. In contrast, patients with cervical intraepithelial neoplasia or cervical cancer present deficient T cell responses [54].

4.3. Mechanisms of HPV to evade the immune system

HPV can be detected and eliminated by an efficient immune system. However, HPV also possess strategies to reduce the actions of the immune system. The best way to trick the immune system is to avoid detection. HPV infects tissues where immune surveillance is limited. In the epithelium of the cervix, the number of DCs greatly declines toward the external layers. Also, the virus replication is coupled with the differentiation state of the infected keratinocyte. Expression of viral proteins increases progressively with differentiation and upward migration of keratinocytes. Thus, the most immunogenic viral proteins are expressed last, in cells that are found in areas of poor immune surveillance (**Figures 3** and **4**). In addition, new virions are released through the normal rupture of surface epithelium. This action prevents inflammation and reduces the virus uptake by DCs. Therefore, HPV replication is a local phenomenon with minimal activation of the immune system.

In addition, HPV has other strategies that interfere with the immune response [27]. The E6 and E7 proteins block IFN production by the infected cell. E6 blocks the transcription factor IFR-3, which activates β-IFN gene expression. With less interferon produced, many interferon-responsive genes are downregulated [55]. Similarly, E7 also inhibits the expression of α-IFN-responsive genes [56, 57]. Also these two oncoproteins can reduce expression of Toll-like receptor (TLR) 9 [58], and some cytokines, such as IL-8 and IL-18 [59, 60]. TLR 9 is expressed in endosomal vesicles where it binds to unmethylated CpG sequences in viral DNA. TLR 9 then signals for production of anti-virus proteins, such as type-I interferon [58]. IL-8 is a potent chemoattractant for neutrophils and T lymphocytes [59], whereas IL-18 induces γ-IFN production by leukocytes [60]. Thus, E6 and E7 proteins can block several innate immune responses. In addition, the viral proteins E5, E6, and E7 can inhibit the expression of MHC class I molecules, reducing recognition of the HPV-infected cell by NK cells and by specific CTLs [61].

5. Prophylactic vaccines

Due to the strong correlation between the presence of HPV infection and tumors, it was thought that by preventing HPV infections, the HPV-induced cancers would disappear. Also as mentioned above, because HPV capsid proteins are recognized by antibodies from infected patients, it is clear that antibodies can bind virus particles. Thus, HPV vaccines that would induce the production of antibodies and could prevent infection were developed in the last decade. The pharmaceutical companies, Merck in the USA and GlaxoSmithKline (GSK) in Europe, created the two prophylactic vaccines approved and used today. Both vaccines, take advantage of the fact that capsid L1 proteins spontaneously assemble in virus-like particles (VLP) without viral DNA. These VLP, produced by overexpressing HPV L1 protein in yeast or insect cells, provide a source of the immunogenic L1 proteins in a non-infective form.

5.1. Cervarix® and Gardasil®

Cervarix® (GSK) is a bivalent vaccine against VLP of HPV types 16 and 18, produced in insect cells [62], whereas Gardasil® (Merck) is a quadrivalent vaccine made with VLP of HPV types

6, 11, 16, and 18, produced in yeast [63]. Both prophylactic vaccines are designed for HPV naïve individuals, since as mentioned above antibodies do not have a protective effect on already infected individuals. These vaccines generate a good antibody response that prevents new infections with high efficacy [64–66] from the HPV types included in the vaccines. Due to a small cross-reactivity [64], these vaccines also show some prophylactic effect on other HPV subtypes not included in the vaccine [67, 68]. However, for the most part these vaccines are effective only for those HPV types included. A new version of these vaccines including nine different types of HPV (6, 11, 16, 18, 31, 33, 45, 52, and 58) has also been developed. Since Gardasil 9® seems to be cost effective compared to the previous vaccines [69], it has also been licensed for clinical use [70].

These vaccines promise to reduce, in the future (30 years from now) the incidence of infection from the HPV types included in them [71]. However, this promise could only be possible if more than 50% of uninfected people get vaccinated. Unfortunately, this kind of coverage for boys and girls before the onset sexual activity, will be difficult and expensive in many parts of the world [72]. Thus, incidence of HPV-related diseases can increase despite HPV vaccination [73] due to many unvaccinated people, who will remain at a high risk and in need for treatment. In addition, distribution of HPV types among cervical malignancies changes all over the world [74–76]. Although, the high-risk HPV 16 and 18 are associated with most cervical cancers in Occident, this is not the case in Asia, where less than 60% of cervical cancer are related to these HPV types [28]. Therefore, the current prophylactic vaccines cannot cover all oncogenic types of HPV in different populations, and their general use in other parts of the world is questionable [68].

5.2. Limitations of current vaccines

As already mentioned, the current prophylactic vaccines against HPV have a limited coverage to only those types included in the vaccine. Since the antibody immune response to L1 proteins is highly specific, no general coverage can be achieved. In addition, the current prophylactic vaccines do not elicit cell-mediated immunity. This means that although these vaccines can protect from most HPV infections (70–80%), the rest of HPV types remain a serious threat for HPV-induced diseases even after vaccination [62, 77]. Despite government efforts to subsidize vaccination programs in order to achieve full coverage, it remains that even vaccinated females must continue cervical cancer screening [78].

These vaccines are directed against the L1 protein of only certain types of HPV. In order to increase coverage vaccines against all HPV types would need to be produced. This will increase the cost of production on multivalent vaccines. The use of adjuvants to augment the immunogenicity of the capsid proteins makes the vaccine thermolabile and also adds to the cost of the vaccine. The problem is that the population that is in need of these vaccines is exactly the one with fewer economical resources. Recently, a two-dose immunization protocol has been tried instead of the recommended three doses schedule. This seems to provide similar protection and thus it is a promising cost reducing strategy [79, 80].

The vaccines are designed for HPV naïve individuals. This requires that very young people get vaccinated before becoming sexually active. The benefit for immunizing older women seems very limited, since no therapeutic effects have been detected for these vaccines [81]. The reason for this is that antibodies induced by these vaccines are directed against the L1 proteins and once the infection is established, these proteins are not expressed. Contrary to this, a therapeutic vaccine would need to be directed against proteins that are expressed throughout the lifecycle of the virus [82] (see next section).

Although, a good humoral immune response is obtained and antibodies are capable of blocking infection, the prevention of cancer by these vaccines is still presumptive. In all clinical trials, the end point has been prevention of only CIN 2/3 lesions. Also, because HPV infections may take a long time to develop cancer, the anti-cancer effect of these vaccines will be known in the future, when vaccinated people become adults and are exposed to the virus [83].

5.3. New prophylactic vaccines

Both current prophylactic vaccines are based on L1 VLP and are therefore very HPV type specific, thermolabile, and costly. The quest for newer vaccines continues with the aim of making them more affordable, more thermostable, and with more coverage toward larger number of HPV types. With these goals in mind, newer prophylactic vaccines are in development. Two kinds are worth mentioning, a L2 protein-based vaccine and a capsomere vaccine.

The capsid L1 protein is highly specific for each type of HPV. In contrast, the L2 protein contains a region that is highly conserved among most high-risk HPV types. This fragment between amino acids 20 and 38 is capable of inducing antibodies that are neutralizing for many HPVs [84]. Unfortunately, the L2 protein is not very immunogenic, and several approaches are being used trying to increase its immunogenicity. These include producing a recombinant protein in bacteria, an expression system in *Lactobacillus casei* for possible oral immunization, and production of L2 VLP derived from bacteriophage PP7 [82, 85].

A VLP formed with L1 protein requires 360 copies of the protein. Thus, a VLP is complex, more expensive to produce, and thermolabile. In contrast, a capsomere is much simpler, thermostable, and cheaper to produce. A capsomere is the basic component of the virus capsid. It has only five L1 copies of the protein, presents similar immunogenicity than an L1 VLP, and can be produced in bacteria [70]. A phase II clinical trial for a HPV 16 L1 capsomere vaccine is currently being conducted (NCT 01355823) [82, 86].

6. Therapeutic vaccines

Preventive vaccines are directed to the external proteins of the virus. By inducing a strong humoral immune response, the antibodies formed can bind to the virus capsid and block the interaction of the virus with endothelial cells. These antibodies can then neutralize the virus and prevent infection. However, this mechanism is not effective when the virus has already entered the cell. Antibodies induced by prophylactic vaccines cannot treat existing viral infections or established HPV-related diseases. Therefore, as discussed above, a high prevalence and mortality of cervical cancer still remains a serious health problem in the world, especially in developing countries [3, 76]. In order to treat an established disease, the elements of the virus present during replication should be the target of the therapy involved. Also, since there are not anti-viral drugs, an effective treatment should be able to stimulate the immune system for elimination of virus-infected cells. An ideal therapeutic vaccine must activate both CD4+ (helper) and CD8+ (cytotoxic) T cells for elimination of the virus [37]. Cytotoxic cells need to recognize a viral antigen expressed in the infected cells. In the case of HPV, the capsid proteins L1 and L2 are expressed in terminally differentiated keratinocytes on the external part of the epithelium; a segment of the tissue where antibodies and cells cannot easily reach (**Figure 2**). In contrast, HPV early proteins, such as E1, E2, E6, and E7, are expressed in multiple stages of the virus infection (**Figure 2**). Consequently, these proteins are all good therapeutic targets.

E2 is a DNA-binding protein involved in activation or repression of different HPV promoters [35], and it also has a relevant role in controlling migration of viral DNA to daughter cells during mitosis of infected cells [87]. Due to these functions, E2 is expressed in all stages of the infection (**Figure 2**). Thus, it is an excellent target for stimulating the immune system for elimination of infected cells at multiple replication stages. In earlier studies, dogs, immunized against papilloma E1 and E2 proteins, did not show papilloma growth after viral challenge, or even presented complete regression of papilloma [88, 89]. These encouraging findings led to devise new vaccines that could activate cellular immune responses to the E2 protein. Clinical trials with these new vaccines have provided very encouraging results (see next section) [90, 91]. As indicated before, the E6 and E7 proteins are important for cancer. Therefore, they are also studied as probable antigens of therapeutic vaccines.

Different types of therapeutic vaccines have been designed and some have also been tested in clinical trials. These novel therapeutic vaccines can be grouped into five categories: peptide-based, protein-based, DNA vaccination, viral vectors, and dendritic cell-based immunization [44, 82]and are described in the following sections.

6.1. Peptide-based vaccines

Instead of using a whole protein, fragments of it can be prepared for immunization. Peptides are cost-effective and safe, but they are also usually poorly immunogenic. Thus, in general, peptides need to be mixed with adjuvants to improve their immunogenicity, deciding what peptides are useful is not easy, however. Recognizing what parts of an HPV antigen are immunogenic is almost impossible to predict and small peptides normally only present linear epitopes. Conformational epitomes that may be needed for an efficient immune response are usually not included. Thus, current preparations contain mixtures of peptides. In addition, because MHC molecules (HLA in humans) are polymorphic, it is possible that some peptides cannot be presented in some patients. An approach used to avoid this, has been the use of restricted HLA-binding peptides. Identification of these peptides is an even more complicated task, making the peptide approach unreliable and more expensive. Also, another complication with this strategy is that exogenously added peptides may load onto MHC class I molecules on cells other than antigen-presenting cells. In this case, the peptide-based vaccine may induce tolerance instead of stimulation [92]. In consequence, the best approach seems to be the use of long overlapping peptides, which appear to be processed and presented correctly by dendritic cells [93].

Despite these complications, some peptide-based vaccines have been tried. In phases I–II clinical trial, one vaccine made of two HPV E7 peptides and one T cell helper peptide, stimulated proliferation of T cells, but it did not induce cytotoxicity against E7 peptides [94]. In a different study, a mixture of long peptides from oncoproteins E6 and E7 in incomplete Freund's adjuvant, was administered to 20 patients with HPV 16-positive, high-grade vulvar intraepithelial neoplasia. In five patients, a T cell response was detected, together with complete regression [95].

Another vaccine (HPV 16-SLP) made of a mixture of long peptides from E6 and E7 proteins, has also been tested. In a group of patients with resected HPV 16-positive cervical cancer, this vaccine induced some HPV 16-specific T cell immune responses including γ-IFN-producing CD4+ T cells. Unfortunately, proliferation of T cells with a regulatory phenotype (Treg) was also detected, suggesting that the response against HPV was not completely effective [96]. In another group of women with high-grade cervical squamous intraepithelial lesions, this vaccine did not induce infiltration of HPV 16-specific T cells into the lesions or HPV clearance [97]. In a third group of patients with HPV 16-positive advanced or recurrent gynecological carcinoma, this vaccine was given with the adjuvant Montanide ISA-51. In this case, a T cell response was detected, but unfortunately no tumor regression or prevention of progressive disease were found [98].

6.2. Protein-based vaccines

Immunization with complete HPV proteins seems a more efficient approach. HPV recombinant proteins can be produced in large quantities and they would provide all possible epitopes of the protein, after processing by APC. However, complete protein still present low immunogenicity and they need to be mixed with adjuvants, or fused to other proteins with more immunogenicity. Some HPV protein vaccines consist of E6 and E7 proteins fused to immunogenic proteins as described next.

A chimeric protein made from the carboxyl-terminally part of HPV 16 L1 protein fused to the amino-terminal part of the HPV 16 E7 protein was produced. This recombinant fusion protein self-assembles into virus-like particles and it has been named L1VLPE7. In a small group of patients with HPV-induced CIN 2/3 lesions, these chimeric VLPs induced antibodies with high titers against HPV L1 and with low titers against HPV E7. Thus, the antibody response again was better toward the capsid protein than the early-gene protein. Consequently, no histological improvement in lesions was observed [99]. Another similar recombinant HPV 16 L1(ΔN26)-E7(ΔC38) protein also assembles into chimeric VLPs. These chimeric VLPs induced neutralizing antibodies and triggered some cell-mediated immune responses in a murine model of cervical cancer [100].

Another fusion protein (SGN-00101) consisting of a heat shock protein (Hsp) from *Mycobacterium bovis* and HPV 16 E7 protein, was administered to patients with CIN 3. Regression to CIN 1was seen in some patients, but it was not clear whether this result was caused by the vaccine or it was just natural regression [101]. Later, the same preparation was administered in several doses during 3 weeks. With this procedure, one-third of patients presented regression that correlated with immune response [102].

Yet, another fusion protein (HPV16 E6/E7) formed by HPV E6 and E7 was produced and tried mixed with the adjuvant ISCOMATRIX. In a group of patients with CIN, this preparation induced a cellular immune response. Unfortunately, the elimination of lesions detected in few patients did not correlate to this immune response [103].

Another recombinant fusion protein made of E6, E7, and L2 proteins (TA-CIN—tissue antigen-cervical intraepithelial neoplasia) has been given to a small group of patients with anogenital intraepithelial neoplasia (AGIN). Unfortunately, there was not a correlation between induction of systemic immunity and clinical outcome [104]. In another group of patients with vulvar intraepithelial neoplasia, a topical application of the immunomodulator, Imiquimod was given for 8 weeks before three doses of TA-CIN at 4-week interval were administered. With this protocol, an important local infiltration of CD8+ and CD4+ T cells in lesions of responding patients was detected, suggesting that the inflammatory state induced by Imiquimod enhances the immune response. Unfortunately, the therapeutic effect was only detected in few patients [105].

6.3. DNA-based vaccines

Another approach for immunization is the use of plasmid DNA coding for the protein of interest. It is known that plasmid DNA, when injected into the skin or muscle can induce immune responses to encoded antigens. The mechanism is poorly understood, and the response is rather inefficient. Yet, new physical methods for delivering DNA seem to induce better immune responses [106]. Some DNA preparations for HPV early proteins have been tried.

A DNA plasmid that encodes for HPV consensus E6/E7 fusion gene (pConE6E7) has been tested in mice and rhesus monkeys. Immunization induced a potent cellular immune response against both E6 and E7 proteins [107], and it was able to delay the growth of established HPV-tumors [108]. Another plasmid encoding E7-specific CTL epitopes from HPV 16 and 18 and embedded in biodegradable micro particles (ZYC101a) was tested in a group of patients histologically confirmed CIN 2/3 neoplasia. About 43% of patients presented regression, compared to 27% of patients receiving placebo, but the difference was not statistically significant, and no correlation between cytotoxic activity and clinical outcome was detected [109]. Another DNA preparation (Amolimogene) contains an encapsulated plasmid encoding some proteins of HPV. In a small group of patients with HPV-associated high-grade CIN, no correlation between cellular immunity and clinical response was reported [110]. Another DNA preparation (Sig-E7(detox)-HSP70) encoding a fusion protein between HPV E7 protein and heat shock protein 70 was tried in a small group of patients with HPV-induced CIN 2/3. Weak HPV E7-specific T cell responses were detected, but not correlation was found between this immune response and clinical outcome [111]. Although DNA vaccines are good tools to enhance the immune system, their approval from regulatory agencies seems unlikely. Regulatory agencies require that novel vaccines fulfill the followings requirements: laboratory demonstration of proof of concept, design end establishment of the manufacturing process, adequate quality and non-clinical safety, clinical trial approval, safety and efficacy, and a marketing authorization application. The use of naked DNA in humans remains a major safety concern, and DNA vaccines, so far have not shown good activation of a specific cellular immune response.

6.4. Recombinant virus

Another approach that has shown better results for treatment of HPV-induced lesions is the use of recombinant viruses. A virus can deliver gene products directly into cells and because an active viral infection takes place, the immune system responds better activating the cellular effector functions. The highly attenuated poxvirus strain modified vaccinia virus Ankara (MVA) has become the vector of choice for novel HPV therapeutic vaccines [112]. This MVA virus is a non-replicating derivative from the virus of the smallpox vaccine. This exceptionally successful vaccine was given to millions of people without any complications. Thus the use of MVA in humans is completely safe. Other advantages of MVA are that it is genetically stable, very immunogenic, and easy to manufacture [113, 114]. The MVA immunogenic potential for cytotoxic responses is due in part to uptake of dying vaccinia virus-infected cells by antigen-presenting cells and cross-presentation of antigens to CD8+ T cells [115]. Several MVA vectors against various diseases are now being evaluated in phase I/II clinical trials [116]. The MVA vectors designed for treatment of HPV are described in the following section.

TA-HPV is a vaccinia virus encoding modified versions of the E6 and E7 genes from HPV 16 and HPV 18. Patients with high-grade vulval intraepithelial neoplasia were immunized intramuscularly with TA-HPV. Some of these (42%) patients presented partial reduction of lesions, but no increase in cytotoxic activity against selected HPV E6 or E7 peptides [117]. In another small group of patients, a partial reduction in lesion diameter, and an infiltration of T cells were observed [118].

Another modified MVA virus contains E6 and E7 proteins together with the human IL-2 gene. This vaccine (TG4001) was given subcutaneously in three weekly doses to 21 patients with CIN 2/3. About half of patients had some clinical responses 6 months later. However, no immune response was reported [119].

Another MVA recombinant virus (MVA E2), containing the bovine papilloma virus (BPV) E2 protein [120], has been has been assessed in several clinical trials. In a group of patients with HPV-induced CIN 1 to CIN 3 lesions, that received MVA E2 injected directly into the uterus once every week for 6 weeks, 94% (34) of patients had complete elimination of precancerous lesions. In addition, an important reduction (90%) in viral DNA load was observed in half of the patients. The others have completely eliminated the virus [90]. Next, in a phase II clinical trial for high-grade lesions, about half (56%) of patients presented complete regression, and in another third (32%) of patients, the lesions were reduced by 90–60% [91]. Importantly, specific cytotoxic activity against cancer cells correlated with clinical outcome [91]. More recently, in a phase III clinical trial, 1176 female patients with anogenital intraepithelial lesions were treated with MVA E2. Most of the patients (89%) showed complete elimination of lesions, and generated a specific cytotoxic response against HPV-transformed cells [121]. These clinical results indicate that MVA E2 is one of the most promising vaccines for therapy of HPV-induced malignancies.

MVA-E1 is a new MVA-based vaccine against HPV. This vaccine consists of the MVA vector encoding the E1 sequence of HPV 16. In a mouse model, immunization with MVA-E1 resulted in sustained HPV E1-specific cellular cytotoxic response [122].

6.5. Dendritic cell-based vaccines

As discussed earlier, dendritic cells (DCs) are major antigen-presenting cells that can efficiently activate cellular immune responses. Based on this, another approach to develop a therapeutic vaccine is the use of dendritic cells pulsed with HPV antigens. The idea is to generate DCs *in vitro* from monocytes taken from the same patient. Then, these DCs are presented with recombinant HPV proteins. The cells should process and present antigens on their membrane. Finally, the pulsed DCs are administered back to the patient to stimulate the immune system. The procedure is complex, time consuming, very costly, and has to be performed individually for each patient.

Earlier studies showed that autologous DCs loaded with HPV E7 protein could induce *in vitro* a specific T cell responses [123], and T cell proliferative responses *in vivo*, [124]. Another study found E7-specific γ-IFN secreting CD8+ T cells in patients treated with autologous DCs pulsed with HPV E7 [125], or with HPV E7 protein and keyhole limpet hemocyanin (KLH) [126]. These reports indicated that DC-based immunization improves T cell responses, but they did not evaluate the therapeutic potential. Recently, it was reported that DCs can be pulsed more efficiently if HPV antigens are directed toward the co-stimulatory molecule CD40 [127]. With a prototype vaccine (anti-CD40-HPV16.E6/7) consisting of a recombinant fusion protein of anti-human CD40 and HPV16 E6/7 protein), DCs could efficiently activate *in vitro* HPV E6/7-specific CD8+ T cells, from the blood of HPV16+ head-and-neck cancer patients [127].

These results show that this approach may be useful in the future if important questions still remaining on the nature and function of dendritic cells can be resolved. For example, are there any unique cell surface receptors that would allow for specific selection of DCs? What are the special DC subsets that can enhance the efficacy of vaccines? What are the DC activators that allow differentiation and/or maturation of a particular type of DC with the ability to promote effector T cells against tumors? Today, DCs are generated *in vitro* from peripheral blood monocytes. This procedure generates cells that vary greatly in their functional capacity, thus making their use in the clinical setting very uncertain.

7. Conclusion

Human papillomavirus (HPV) infections remain an important public health issue because they are associated to cervical carcinoma, the second most common cancer among women [4]. Two preventive vaccines have been approved and promise to achieve in the future, a reduction in HPV-related cancer incidence. However, these vaccines are not the complete solution. Since complete vaccination coverage is difficult and costly in many parts of the world [72], and since these vaccines are highly HPV type specific, only the high-risk HPV types responsible for about 60% of all cervical cancers (HPV 16 and 18) are included in these preventive vaccines, a large population will remain at a high risk of HPV infections. Also, these preventive vaccines do not have any therapeutic potential. Therefore, many people remain in need of efficient treatment for HPV-related diseases.

Novel therapeutic vaccines for treatment of HPV-infected tissues are now being tested for their potential to activate an immune cellular response. Different types of therapeutic vaccines are considered. Studies, so far have shown variable results for most of them. However, the therapeutic vaccines using recombinant virus have demonstrated to be very effective in clinical settings. Thus, recombinant vaccinia therapies are today the most promising candidates for a successful treatment of HPV-induced cancers.

Acknowledgements

The research in the authors' laboratories is supported by Virolab, S de RL de CV, and by grant 254434 (to CR) from Consejo Nacional de Ciencia y Tecnología, Mexico.

Author details

Carlos Rosales[1] and Ricardo Rosales[2]*

*Address all correspondence to: rrosalesvirolab10@gmail.com

1 Immunology Department, Instituto de Investigaciones Biomédicas, Universidad Nacional Autónoma de México, Mexico City, Mexico

2 Virolab, S de RL de CV, Cuernavaca, Morelos, Mexico

References

[1] Jablonska S, Dabrowski J, Jakubowicz K. Epidermodysplasia verruciformis as a model in studies on the role of papovaviruses in oncogenesis. Cancer Research. 1972;**32**:583-589

[2] zur Hausen H, de Villiers EM, Gissmann L. Papillomavirus infections and human genital cancer. Gynecologic Oncology. 1981;**12**:S124-S128

[3] Forman D, de Martel C, Lacey CJ, Soerjomataram I, Lortet-Tieulent J, Bruni L, Vignat J, Ferlay J, Bray F, Plummer M, et al. Global burden of human papillomavirus and related diseases. Vaccine. 2012;**30**:F12-F23. DOI: 10.1016/j.vaccine.2012.07.055

[4] Arbyn M, Castellsagué X, de Sanjosé S, Bruni L, Saraiya M, Bray F, Ferlay J. Worldwide burden of cervical cancer in 2008. Annals of Oncology. 2011;**22**:2675-2686. DOI: 10.1093/annonc/mdr015

[5] Egawa N, Egawa K, Griffin H, Doorbar J. Human papillomaviruses; epithelial tropisms, and the development of neoplasia. Viruses. 2015;**7**:3863-3890. DOI: 10.3390/v7072802

[6] Bernard HU. Taxonomy and phylogeny of papillomaviruses: An overview and recent developments. Infection, Genetics and Evolution. 2013;**18**:357-361. DOI: 10.1016/j.meegid.2013.03.011

[7] Lacey CJ, Lowndes CM, Shah KV. Chapter 4: Burden and management of non-cancerous HPV-related conditions: HPV-6/11 disease. Vaccine. 2006;**24**(Suppl 3):S3/35-S33/41

[8] Muñoz N, Bosch FX. The causal link between HPV and cervical cancer and its implications for prevention of cervical cancer. Bulletin of the Pan American Health Organization. 1996;**30**:362-367

[9] Parkin DM, Bray F. Chapter 2: The burden of HPV-related cancers. Vaccine. 2006;**24**: S11-S25

[10] D'Souza G, Fakhry C, Sugar EA, Seaberg EC, Weber K, Minkoff HL, Anastos K, Palefsky JM, Gillison ML. Six-month natural history of oral versus cervical human papillomavirus infection. International Journal of Cancer. 2007;**121**:143-150

[11] Cantley RL, Gabrielli E, Montebelli F, Cimbaluk D, Gattuso P, Petruzzelli G. Ancillary studies in determining human papillomavirus status of squamous cell carcinoma of the oropharynx: A review. Pathology Research International. 2011;**2011**:138469. DOI: 10.4061/2011/138469

[12] Herberhold S, Hellmich M, Panning M, Bartok E, Silling S, Akgül B, Wieland U. Human polyomavirus and human papillomavirus prevalence and viral load in non-malignant tonsillar tissue and tonsillar carcinoma. Medical Microbiology and Immunology. 2016;Nov 10;**206**. [Epub ahead of print]. DOI: 10.1007/s00430-016-0486-6

[13] Schiffman M, Castle PE, Jeronimo J, Rodriguez AC, Wacholder S. Human papillomavirus and cervical cancer. Lancet. 2007;**370**:890-907

[14] Woodman CB, Collins SI, Young LS. The natural history of cervical HPV infection: Unresolved issues. Nature Reviews Cancer. 2007;**7**:11-22

[15] Ghittoni R, Accardi R, Chiocca S, Tommasino M. Role of human papillomaviruses in carcinogenesis. Ecancermedicalscience. 2015;**9**:526. DOI: 10.3332/ecancer.2015.526

[16] Trimble CL, Piantadosi S, Gravitt P, Ronnett B, Pizer E, Elko A, Wilgus B, Yutzy W, Daniel R, Shah K, et al. Spontaneous regression of high-grade cervical dysplasia: Effects of human papillomavirus type and HLA phenotype. Clinical Cancer Research. 2005;**11**:4717-4723

[17] Nuovo GJ, Friedman D, Richart RM. In situ hybridization analysis of human papillomavirus DNA segregation patterns in lesions of the female genital tract. Gynecologic Oncology. 1990;**36**:256-262

[18] Cuzick J, Bergeron C, von Knebel DM, Gravitt P, Jeronimo J, Lorincz AT, J L M Meijer C, Sankaranarayanan R, J F Snijders P, Szarewski A. New technologies and procedures for cervical cancer screening. Vaccine. 2012;**30**:F107-F116. DOI: 10.1016/j.vaccine.2012.05.088

[19] Poljak M, Cuzick J, Kocjan BJ, Iftner T, Dillner J, Arbyn M. Nucleic acid tests for the detection of alpha human papillomaviruses. Vaccine. 2012;**30**:F100-F106. DOI: 10.1016/j.vaccine.2012.04.105

[20] Solomon D, Davey D, Kurman R, Moriarty A, O'Connor D, Prey M, Raab S, Sherman M, Wilbur D, Wright TJ, et al. The 2001 Bethesda System: Terminology for reporting results of cervical cytology. JAMA. 2002;**287**:2114-2119

[21] American Cancer Society. Survival Rates for Cancer of the Cervix. 2013. http://www.cancer.org/cancer/cervicalcancer/overviewguide/cervical-cancer-overview-survival-rates

[22] Hajj Hussein I, Chams N, Chams S, El Sayegh S, Badran R, Raad M, Gerges-Geagea A, Leone A, Jurjus A. Vaccines through centuries: Major cornerstones of global health. Frontiers in Public Health. 2015;**3**:269. DOI: 10.3389/fpubh.2015.00269

[23] Kash N, Lee MA, Kollipara R, Downing C, Guidry J, Tyring SK. Safety and efficacy data on vaccines and immunization to human papillomavirus. Journal of Clinical Medicine. 2015;**4**:614-633. DOI: 10.3390/jcm4040614

[24] Harper DM. Current prophylactic HPV vaccines and gynecologic premalignancies. Current Opinion in Obstetrics & Gynecology. 2009;**21**:457-464. DOI: 10.1097/GCO.0b013e328332c910

[25] Harper DM, Williams KB. Prophylactic HPV vaccines: Current knowledge of impact on gynecologic premalignancies. Discovery Medicine. 2010;**10**:7-17

[26] Ma B, Maraj B, Tran NP, Knoff J, Chen A, Alvarez RD, Hung CF, Wu TC. Emerging human papillomavirus vaccines. Expert Opinion on Emerging Drugs. 2012;**17**:469-492. DOI: 10.1517/14728214.2012.744393

[27] Stanley M. Immune responses to human papillomavirus. Vaccine 2006;**30**:S16-S22

[28] Kawana K, Adachi K, Kojima S, Kozuma S, Fujii T. Therapeutic human papillomavirus (HPV) vaccines: A novel approach. The Open Virology Journal. 2012;**6**:264-269. DOI: 10.2174/1874357901206010264

[29] Stern PL, van der Burg SH, Hampson IN, Broker TR, Fiander A, Lacey CJ, Kitchener HC, Einstein MH. Therapy of human papillomavirus-related disease. Vaccine. 2012;**30**:F71-F82. DOI: 10.1016/j.vaccine.2012.05.091

[30] Doorbar J, Quint W, Banks L, Bravo IG, Stoler M, Broker TR, Stanley MA. The biology and life-cycle of human papillomaviruses. Vaccine. 2012;**30**:F55-F70. DOI: 10.1016/j.vaccine.2012.06.083

[31] Doorbar J. Latent papillomavirus infections and their regulation. Current Opinion in Virology. 2013;**3**:416-421. DOI: 10.1016/j.coviro.2013.06.003

[32] Titolo S, Pelletier A, Sauvé F, Brault K, Wardrop E, White PW, Amin A, Cordingley MG, Archambault J. Role of the ATP-binding domain of the human papillomavirus type 11 E1 helicase in E2-dependent binding to the origin. Journal of Virology. 1999;**73**:5282-5293

[33] Titolo S, Pelletier A, Pulichino AM, Brault K, Wardrop E, White PW, Cordingley MG, Archambault J. Identification of domains of the human papillomavirus type 11 E1 helicase involved in oligomerization and binding to the viral origin. Journal of Virology. 2000;**74**:7349-7361

[34] Hegde RS. The papillomavirus E2 proteins: Structure, function, and biology. Annual Review of Biophysics and Biomolecular Structure. 2002;**31**:343-360

[35] McBride AA. The papillomavirus E2 proteins. Virology. 2013;**445**:57-79. DOI: 10.1016/j.virol.2013.06.006

[36] Stern PL, Einstein MH. From HPV infection to oncogenesis: A brief review of the complex immunobiological events. Current Cancer Therapy Reviews. 2010;**6**:110-116

[37] Best SR, Niparko KJ, Pai SI. Biology of HPV infection and immune therapy for HPV-related head and neck cancers. Otolaryngologic Clinics of North America. 2012;**45**:807-822. DOI:10.1016/j.otc.2012.04.005

[38] Doorbar J. The E4 protein; structure, function and patterns of expression. Virology. 2013;**445**:80-98. DOI: 10.1016/j.virol.2013.07.008

[39] DiMaio D, Petti LM. The E5 proteins. Virology. 2013;**445**:99-114. DOI: 10.1016/j.virol.2013.05.006

[40] Buck CB, Day PM, Trus BL. The papillomavirus major capsid protein L1. Virology. 2013;**445**:169-174. DOI: 10.1016/j.virol.2013.05.038

[41] Buck CB, Cheng N, Thompson CD, Lowy DR, Steven AC, Schiller JT, Trus BL. Arrangement of L2 within the papillomavirus capsid. Journal of Virological Methods. 2008;**82**:5190-5197. DOI: 10.1128/JVI.02726-07

[42] Buck CB, Thompson CD, Pang YY, Lowy DR, Schiller JT. Maturation of papillomavirus capsids. Journal of Virology. 2005;**79**:2839-2846

[43] von Krogh G, Lacey CJ, Gross G, Barrasso R, Schneider A. European course on HPV associated pathology: Guidelines for primary care physicians for the diagnosis and management of anogenital warts. Sexually Transmitted Infections. 2000;**76**:162-168

[44] Rosales R, Rosales C. Immune therapy for human papillomaviruses-related cancers. World Journal of Clinical Oncology. 2014;**5**:1002-1019. DOI: 10.5306/wjco.v5.i5.1002

[45] Sonnex C, Lacey CJ. The treatment of human papillomavirus lesions of the lower genital tract. Best Practice & Research. Clinical Obstetrics & Gynaecology. 2001;**15**:801-816

[46] Woodworth CD. HPV innate immunity. Frontiers in Bioscience. 2002;**7**:2058-2071

[47] Degli-Esposti MA, Smyth MJ. Close encounters of different kinds: Dendritic cells and NK cells take centre stage. Nature Reviews Immunology. 2005;**5**:112-124

[48] Zhang N, Bevan MJ. CD8(+) T cells: Foot soldiers of the immune system. Immunity. 2011;**35**:161-168. DOI: 10.1016/j.immuni.2011.07.010

[49] Bourgault Villada I, Moyal Barracco M, Ziol M, Chaboissier A, Barget N, Berville S, Paniel B, Jullian E, Clerici T, Maillère B, et al. Spontaneous regression of grade 3 vulvar intraepithelial neoplasia associated with human papillomavirus-16-specific CD4(+) and CD8(+) T-cell responses. Cancer Research. 2004;**64**:8761-8766

[50] Paternoster DM, Cester M, Resente C, Pascoli I, Nanhorngue K, Marchini F, Boccagni P, Cillo U, Ribaldone R, Amoruso E, et al. Human papillomavirus infection and cervical intraepithelial neoplasia in transplanted patients. Transplantation Proceedings. 2008;**40**:1877-1880. DOI: 10.1016/j.transproceed.2008.05.074

[51] Moscicki AB, Ellenberg JH, Farhat S, Xu J. Persistence of human papillomavirus infection in HIV-infected and -uninfected adolescent girls: Risk factors and differences, by phylogenetic type. The Journal of Infectious Diseases. 2004;**190**:37-45

[52] Tjiong MY, Zumbach K, Schegget JT, van der Vange N, Out TA, Pawlita M, Struyk L. Antibodies against human papillomavirus type 16 and 18 E6 and E7 proteins in cervicovaginal washings and serum of patients with cervical neoplasia. Viral Immunology. 2001;**14**:415-424

[53] Welters MJ, de Jong A, van den Eeden SJ, van der Hulst JM, Kwappenberg KM, Hassane S, Franken KL, Drijfhout JW, Fleuren GJ, Kenter G, et al. Frequent display of human papillomavirus type 16 E6-specific memory t-Helper cells in the healthy population as witness of previous viral encounter. Cancer Research. 2003;**63**:636-641

[54] de Jong A, van Poelgeest MI, van der Hulst JM, Drijfhout JW, Fleuren GJ, Melief CJ, Kenter G, Offringa R, van der Burg SH. Human papillomavirus type 16-positive cervical cancer is associated with impaired CD4+ T-cell immunity against early antigens E2 and E6. Cancer Research. 2004;**64**:5449-5455

[55] Nees M, Geoghegan JM, Hyman T, Frank S, Miller L, Woodworth CD. Papillomavirus type 16 oncogenes downregulate expression of interferon-responsive genes and upregulate proliferation-associated and NF-kappaB-responsive genes in cervical keratinocytes. Journal of Virology. 2001;**75**:4283-4296

[56] Barnard P, Payne E, McMillan NA. The human papillomavirus E7 protein is able to inhibit the antiviral and anti-growth functions of interferon-alpha. Virology. 2000;**277**:411-419

[57] Li S, Labrecque S, Gauzzi MC, Cuddihy AR, Wong AH, Pellegrini S, Matlashewski GJ, Koromilas AE. The human papillomavirus (HPV)-18 E6 oncoprotein physically associates with Tyk2 and impairs Jak-STAT activation by interferon-alpha. Oncogene. 1999;**18**:5727-5737

[58] Hasan UA, Bates E, Takeshita F, Biliato A, Accardi R, Bouvard V, Mansour M, Vincent I, Gissmann L, Iftner T, et al. TLR9 expression and function is abolished by the cervical cancer-associated human papillomavirus type 16. Journal of Immunology. 2007;**178**:3186-3197

[59] Huang SM, McCance DJ. Down regulation of the interleukin-8 promoter by human papillomavirus type 16 E6 and E7 through effects on CREB binding protein/p300 and P/CAF. Journal of Virology. 2002;**76**:8710-8721

[60] Lee SJ, Cho YS, Cho MC, Shim JH, Lee KA, Ko KK, Choe YK, Park SN, Hoshino T, Kim S, et al. Both E6 and E7 oncoproteins of human papillomavirus 16 inhibit IL-18-induced IFN-gamma production in human peripheral blood mononuclear and NK cells. Journal of Immunology. 2001;**167**:497-504

[61] Heller C, Weisser T, Mueller-Schickert A, Rufer E, Hoh A, Leonhardt RM, Knittle MR. Identification of key amino acid residues that determine the ability of high risk HPV16-E7 to dysregulate major histocompatibility complex class I expression. The Journal of Biological Chemistry. 2011;**286**:10983-10997. DOI: 10.1074/jbc.M110.199190

[62] Harper DM, Franco EL, Wheeler CM, Moscicki AB, Romanowski B, Roteli-Martins CM, Jenkins D, Schuind A, Costa Clemens SA, Dubin G, et al. Sustained efficacy up to 4.5 years of a bivalent L1 virus-like particle vaccine against human papillomavirus types 16 and 18: Follow-up from a randomised control trial. Lancet. 2006;**367**:1247-1255

[63] Villa LL, Costa RL, Petta CA, Andrade RP, Paavonen J, Iversen OE, Olsson SE, Høye J, Steinwall M, Riis-Johannessen G, et al. High sustained efficacy of a prophylactic quadrivalent human papillomavirus types 6/11/16/18 L1 virus-like particle vaccine through 5 years of follow-up. British Journal of Cancer. 2006;**95**:1459-1466

[64] Paavonen J, Naud P, Salmerón J, Wheeler CM, Chow SN, Apter D, Kitchener H, Castellsague X, Teixeira JC, Skinner SR, et al. Efficacy of human papillomavirus (HPV)-16/18 AS04-adjuvanted vaccine against cervical infection and precancer caused by oncogenic HPV types (PATRICIA): Final analysis of a double-blind, randomised study in young women. Lancet. 2009;**374**:301-314. DOI: 10.1016/S0140-6736(09)61248-4

[65] Kjaer SK, Sigurdsson K, Iversen OE, Hernandez-Avila M, Wheeler CM, Perez G, Brown DR, Koutsky LA, Tay EH, García P, et al. A pooled analysis of continued prophylactic efficacy of quadrivalent human papillomavirus (Types 6/11/16/18) vaccine against high-grade cervical and external genital lesions. Cancer Prevention Research (Phila). 2009;**2**:868-878. DOI: 10.1158/1940-6207.CAPR-09-0031

[66] FUTURE I/II Study Group, Dillner J, Kjaer SK, Wheeler CM, Sigurdsson K, Iversen OE, Hernandez-Avila M, Perez G, Brown DR, Koutsky LA, et al. Four year efficacy of prophylactic human papillomavirus quadrivalent vaccine against low grade cervical, vulvar, and vaginal intraepithelial neoplasia and anogenital warts: Randomised controlled trial. BMJ. 2010;**341**:c3493. DOI: 10.1136/bmj.c3493

[67] Muñoz N, Kjaer SK, Sigurdsson K, Iversen OE, Hernandez-Avila M, Wheeler CM, Perez G, Brown DR, Koutsky LA, Tay EH, et al. Impact of human papillomavirus (HPV)-6/11/16/18 vaccine on all HPV-associated genital diseases in young women. Journal of the National Cancer Institute. 2010;**102**:325-339. DOI: 10.1093/jnci/djp534

[68] Tomljenovic L, Shaw CA. Human papillomavirus (HPV) vaccine policy and evidence-based medicine: Are they at odds?. Annals of Medicine. 2013;**45**:182-193. DOI: 10.3109/07853890.2011.645353

[69] Drolet M, Laprise JF, Boily MC, Franco EL, Brisson M. Potential cost-effectiveness of the nonavalent human papillomavirus (HPV) vaccine. International Journal of Cancer. 2014;**134**:2264-2268. DOI: 10.1002/ijc.28541

[70] Panatto D, Amicizia D, Bragazzi NL, Rizzitelli E, Tramalloni D, Valle I, Gasparini R. Human papillomavirus vaccine: State of the art and future perspectives. Advances in Protein Chemistry and Structural Biology. 2015;**101**:231-322. DOI: 10.1016/bs.apcsb.2015.08.004

[71] Dillner J, Arbyn M, Unger E, Dillner L. Monitoring of human papillomavirus vaccination. Clinical and Experimental Immunology. 2011;**163**:17-25. DOI: 10.1111/j.1365-2249.2010.04268.x

[72] van Bogaert L. Are the currently existing anti-human papillomavirus vaccines appropriate for the developing world? Annals of Medicine and Health Science Research. 2013;**3**:306-312

[73] Harper DM, Nieminen P, Paavonen J, Lehtinen M. Cervical cancer incidence can increase despite HPV vaccination. The Lancet Infectious Diseases. 2010;**10**:594-595. DOI: 10.1016/S1473-3099(10)70182-1

[74] Clifford GM, Rana RK, Franceschi S, Smith JS, Gough G, Pimenta JM. Human papillomavirus genotype distribution in low-grade cervical lesions: Comparison by geographic region and with cervical cancer. Cancer Epidemiology, Biomarkers & Prevention. 2005;**14**:1157-1164

[75] Smith JS, Lindsay L, Hoots B, Keys J, Franceschi S, Winer R, Clifford GM. Human papillomavirus type distribution in invasive cervical cancer and high-grade cervical lesions: A meta-analysis update. International Journal of Cancer. 2007;**121**:621-632

[76] Husain RS, Ramakrishnan V. Global variation of human papillomavirus genotypes and selected genes involved in cervical malignancies. Annals of Global Health. 2015;**81**:675-683. DOI: 10.1016/j.aogh.2015.08.026

[77] Einstein MH, Schiller JT, Viscidi RP, Strickler HD, Coursaget P, Tan T, Halsey N, Jenkins D. Clinician's guide to human papillomavirus immunology: Knowns and unknowns. The Lancet Infectious Diseases. 2009;**9**:347-356. DOI: 10.1016/S1473-3099(09)70108-2

[78] American Cancer Society. Can Cancer of the Cervix be Prevented?. 2013. http://www.cancer.org/cancer/cervicalcancer/overviewguide/cervical-cancer-overview-prevention

[79] Jit M, Laprise JF, Choi YH, Brisson M. Fewer than three doses of HPV vaccine. The Lancet Oncology. 2015;**16**:e423-e424. DOI: 10.1016/S1470-2045(15)00229-6

[80] Kreimer AR, Struyf F, Del Rosario-Raymundo MR, Hildesheim A, Skinner SR, Wacholder S, Garland SM, Herrero R, David MP, Wheeler CM, et al. Efficacy of fewer than three doses of an HPV-16/18 AS04-adjuvanted vaccine: Combined analysis of data from the Costa Rica Vaccine and PATRICIA trials. The Lancet Oncology. 2015;**16**:775-786. DOI: 10.1016/S1470-2045(15)00047-9

[81] Wang JW, Roden RB. Virus-like particles for the prevention of human papillomavirus-associated malignancies. Expert Review of Vaccines. 2013;**12**:129-141. DOI: 10.1586/erv.12.151

[82] Kumar S, Biswas M, Jose T. HPV vaccine: Current status and future directions. Medical Journal Armed Forces India. 2015;**71**:171-177. DOI: 10.1016/j.mjafi.2015.02.006

[83] Schiller JT, Castellsagué X, Garland SM. A review of clinical trials of human papillomavirus prophylactic vaccines. Vaccine. 2012;**30**:F123-F138. DOI: 10.1016/j.vaccine.2012.04.108

[84] Wang JW, Roden RB. L2, the minor capsid protein of papillomavirus. Virology. 2013;**445**:175-186. DOI: 10.1016/j.virol.2013.04.017

[85] Schellenbacher C, Roden RB, Kirnbauer R. Developments in L2-based human papillomavirus (HPV) vaccines. Virus Research. 2016;**231**:pii: S0168-1702(16)30528-7 [Epub ahead of print]. DOI: 10.1016/j.virusres.2016.11.020

[86] Fraillery D, Baud D, Pang SY, Schiller J, Bobst M, Zosso N, Ponci F, Nardelli-Haefliger D. Salmonella enterica serovar Typhi Ty21a expressing human papillomavirus type 16 L1 as a potential live vaccine against cervical cancer and typhoid fever. Clinical and Vaccine Immunology. 2007;**14**:1285-1295. DOI: 10.1128/CVI.00164-07

[87] Ibeanu OA. Molecular pathogenesis of cervical cancer. Cancer Biology & Therapy. 2011;**11**:295-306

[88] Moore RA, Walcott S, White KL, Anderson DM, Jain S, Lloyd A, Topley P, Thomsen L, Gough GW, Stanley MA. Therapeutic immunisation with COPV early genes by epithelial DNA delivery. Virology. 2003;**314**:630-635

[89] Moore RA, Santos EB, Nicholls PK, White KL, Anderson DM, Lloyd A, Topley P, Romanos M, Thomsen L, Parmar V, et al. Intraepithelial DNA immunisation with a plasmid encoding a codon optimised COPV E1 gene sequence, but not the wild-type gene sequence completely protects against mucosal challenge with infectious COPV in beagles. Virology. 2002;**304**:451-459

[90] Corona-Gutierrez CM, Tinoco A, Navarro T, Contreras ML, Cortes RR, Calzado P, Reyes L, Posternak R, Morosoli G, Verde ML, et al. Therapeutic vaccination with MVA E2 can eliminate precancerous lesions (CIN 1, CIN 2, and CIN 3) associated with infection by oncogenic human papillomavirus. Human Gene Therapy. 2004;**15**:421-431

[91] García-Hernández E, González-Sánchez JL, Andrade-Manzano A, Contreras ML, Padilla S, Guzmán CC, Jiménez R, Reyes L, Morosoli G, Verde ML, et al. Regression of papilloma high-grade lesions (CIN 2 and CIN 3) is stimulated by therapeutic vaccination with MVA E2 recombinant vaccine. Cancer Gene Therapy. 2006;**13**:592-597

[92] Melief CJ, van der Burg SH. Immunotherapy of established (pre)malignant disease by synthetic long peptide vaccines. Nature Reviews Cancer. 2008;**8**:351-360. DOI: 10.1038/nrc2373

[93] Rosalia RA, Quakkelaar ED, Redeker A, Khan S, Camps M, Drijfhout JW, Silva AL, Jiskoot W, van Hall T, van Veelen PA, et al. Dendritic cells process synthetic long peptides better than whole protein, improving antigen presentation and T-cell activation. European Journal of Immunology. 2013;**43**:2554-2565. DOI: 10.1002/eji.201343324

[94] Ressing ME, van Driel WJ, Brandt RM, Kenter GG, de Jong JH, Bauknecht T, Fleuren GJ, Hoogerhout P, Offringa R, Sette A, et al. Detection of T helper responses, but not of human papillomavirus-specific cytotoxic T lymphocyte responses, after peptide vaccination of patients with cervical carcinoma. Journal of Immunotherapy. 2000;**23**:255-266

[95] Kenter GG, Welters MJ, Valentijn AR, Lowik MJ, Berends-van der Meer DM, Vloon AP, Essahsah F, Fathers LM, Offringa R, Drijfhout JW, et al. Vaccination against HPV-16 oncoproteins for vulvar intraepithelial neoplasia. The New England Journal of Medicine. 2009;**361**:1838-1847. DOI: 10.1056/NEJMoa0810097

[96] Welters MJ, Kenter GG, Piersma SJ, Vloon AP, Löwik MJ, Berends-van der Meer DM, Drijfhout JW, Valentijn AR, Wafelman AR, Oostendorp J, et al. Induction of tumor-specific CD4+ and CD8+ T-cell immunity in cervical cancer patients by a human papillomavirus type 16 E6 and E7 long peptides vaccine. Clinical Cancer Research. 2008;**14**:178-187. DOI: 10.1158/1078-0432.CCR-07-1880

[97] de Vos van Steenwijk PJ, Ramwadhdoebe TH, Löwik MJ, van der Minne CE, Berends-van der Meer DM, Fathers LM, Valentijn AR, Oostendorp J, Fleuren GJ, Hellebrekers BW, et al. A placebo-controlled randomized HPV16 synthetic long-peptide vaccination study in women with high-grade cervical squamous intraepithelial lesions. Cancer Immunology. 2012;**61**:1485-1492. DOI: 10.1007/s00262-012-1292-7

[98] van Poelgeest MI, Welters MJ, van Esch EM, Stynenbosch LF, Kerpershoek G, van Persijn van Meerten EL, van den Hende M, Löwik MJ, Berends-van der Meer DM, Fathers LM, et al. HPV16 synthetic long peptide (HPV16-SLP) vaccination therapy of patients with advanced or recurrent HPV16-induced gynecological carcinoma, a phase II trial. Journal of Translational Medicine. 2013;**11**:88. DOI: 10.1186/1479-5876-11-88

[99] Kaufmann AM, Nieland JD, Jochmus I, Baur S, Friese K, Gabelsberger J, Gieseking F, Gissmann L, Glasschröder B, Grubert T, et al. Vaccination trial with HPV16 L1E7 chimeric virus-like particles in women suffering from high grade cervical intraepithelial neoplasia (CIN 2/3). International Journal of Cancer. 2007;**121**:2794-2800

[100] Sharma C, Dey B, Wahiduzzaman M, Singh N. Human papillomavirus 16 L1-E7 chimeric virus like particles show prophylactic and therapeutic efficacy in murine model of cervical cancer. Vaccine. 2012;**30**:5417-5424. DOI: 10.1016/j.vaccine.2012.06.010

[101] Einstein MH, Kadish AS, Burk RD, Kim MY, Wadler S, Streicher H, Goldberg GL, Runowicz CD. Heat shock fusion protein-based immunotherapy for treatment of cervical intraepithelial neoplasia III. Gynecologic Oncology. 2007;**106**:453-460

[102] Roman LD, Wilczynski S, Muderspach LI, Burnett AF, O'Meara A, Brinkman JA, Kast WM, Facio G, Felix JC, Aldana M, et al. A phase II study of Hsp-7 (SGN-00101) in women with high-grade cervical intraepithelial neoplasia. Gynecologic Oncology. 2007;**106**:558-566

[103] Frazer IH, Quinn M, Nicklin JL, Tan J, Perrin LC, Ng P, O'Connor VM, White O, Wendt N, Martin J, et al. Phase 1 study of HPV16-specific immunotherapy with E6E7 fusion protein and ISCOMATRIX adjuvant in women with cervical intraepithelial neoplasia. Vaccine. 2004;**23**:172-181

[104] Smyth LJ, Van Poelgeest MI, Davidson EJ, Kwappenberg KM, Burt D, Sehr P, Pawlita M, Man S, Hickling JK, Fiander AN, et al. Immunological responses in women with human papillomavirus type 16 (HPV-16)-associated anogenital intraepithelial neoplasia induced by heterologous prime-boost HPV-16 oncogene vaccination. Clinical Cancer Research. 2004;**10**:2954-2961

[105] Daayana S, Elkord E, Winters U, Pawlita M, Roden R, Stern PL, Kitchener HC. Phase II trial of imiquimod and HPV therapeutic vaccination in patients with vulval intraepithelial neoplasia. British Journal of Cancer. 2010;**30**:1129-1136. DOI: 10.1038/sj.bjc.6605611

[106] Ferraro B, Morrow MP, Hutnick NA, Shin TH, Lucke CE, Weiner DB. Clinical applications of DNA vaccines: Current progress. Clinical Infectious Diseases. 2011;**53**:296-302. DOI: 10.1093/cid/cir334

[107] Yan J, Harris K, Khan AS, Draghia-Akli R, Sewell D, Weiner DB. Cellular immunity induced by a novel HPV18 DNA vaccine encoding an E6/E7 fusion consensus protein in mice and rhesus macaques. Vaccine 2008;**26**:5210-5215. DOI: 10.1016/j.vaccine.2008.03.069

[108] Yan J, Reichenbach DK, Corbitt N, Hokey DA, Ramanathan MP, McKinney KA, Weiner DB, Sewell D. Induction of antitumor immunity *in vivo* following delivery of a novel HPV-16 DNA vaccine encoding an E6/E7 fusion antigen. Vaccine. 2009;**27**:431-440. DOI: 10.1016/j.vaccine.2008.10.078

[109] Garcia F, Petry KU, Muderspach L, Gold MA, Braly P, Crum CP, Magill M, Silverman M, Urban RG, Hedley ML, et al. ZYC101a for treatment of high-grade cervical intraepithelial neoplasia: A randomized controlled trial. Obstetrics and Gynecology. 2004;**103**:317-326

[110] Matijevic M, Hedley ML, Urban RG, Chicz RM, Lajoie C, Luby TM. Immunization with a poly (lactide co-glycolide) encapsulated plasmid DNA expressing antigenic regions of HPV 16 and 18 results in an increase in the precursor frequency of T cells that respond to epitopes from HPV 16, 18, 6 and 11. Cellular Immunology. 2011;**270**:62-69. DOI: 10.1016/j.cellimm.2011.04.005

[111] Trimble CL, Peng S, Kos F, Gravitt P, Viscidi R, Sugar E, Pardoll D, Wu TC. A phase I trial of a human papillomavirus DNA vaccine for HPV16+ cervical intraepithelial neoplasia 2/3. Clinical Cancer Research. 2009;**15**:361-367. DOI: 10.1158/1078-0432.CCR-08-1725

[112] Su JH, Wu A, Scotney E, Ma B, Monie A, Hung CF, Wu TC. Immunotherapy for cervical cancer: Research status and clinical potential. BioDrugs. 2010;**24**:109-129. DOI: 10.2165/11532810-000000000-00000

[113] Gilbert SC. Clinical development of modified vaccinia virus ankara vaccines. Vaccine 2013;**31**:4241-4246. DOI: 10.1016/j.vaccine.2013.03.020

[114] Cottingham MG, Carroll MW. Recombinant MVA vaccines: Dispelling the myths. Vaccine. 2013;**31**:4247-4251. DOI: 10.1016/j.vaccine.2013.03.021

[115] Iborra S, Izquierdo HM, Martínez-López M, Blanco-Menéndez N, Reis e Sousa C, Sancho D. The DC receptor DNGR-1 mediates cross-priming of CTLs during vaccinia virus infection in mice. The Journal of Clinical Investigation. 2012;**122**:1628-1643. DOI: 10.1172/JCI60660

[116] Gómez CE, Perdiguero B, García-Arriaza J, Esteban M. Clinical applications of attenuated MVA poxvirus strain. Expert Review of Vaccines. 2013;**12**:1395-1416. DOI: 10.1586/14760584.2013.845531

[117] Baldwin PJ, van der Burg SH, Boswell CM, Offringa R, Hickling JK, Dobson J, Roberts JS, Latimer JA, Moseley RP, Coleman N, et al. Vaccinia-expressed human papillomavirus 16 and 18 e6 and e7 as a therapeutic vaccination for vulval and vaginal intraepithelial neoplasia. Clinical Cancer Research. 2003;**9**:5205-5213

[118] Davidson EJ, Boswell CM, Sehr P, Pawlita M, Tomlinson AE, McVey RJ, Dobson J, Roberts JS, Hickling J, Kitchener HC, et al. Immunological and clinical responses in women with vulval intraepithelial neoplasia vaccinated with a vaccinia virus encoding human papillomavirus 16/18 oncoproteins. Cancer Research. 2003;**63**:6032-6041

[119] Brun J-L, Dalstein V, Leveque J, Mathevet P, Raulic P, Baldauf JJ, Scholl S, Huynh B, Douvier S, Riethmuller D, et al. Regression of high-grade cervical intraepithelial neoplasia with TG4001 targeted immunotherapy. American Journal of Obstetrics and Gynecology. 2011;**204**:169.e161-169.e168. DOI: 10.1016/j.ajog.2010.09.020

[120] Rosales C, Valadez-Graham V, Rosas GA, Merchant H, Rosales R. A recombinant vaccinia virus containing the papilloma E2 protein promotes tumor regression by stimulating macrophage antibody-dependent cytotoxicity. Cancer Immunology. 2000;**49**:347-360

[121] Rosales R, López-Contreras M, Rosales C, Magallanes-Molina J-R, Gonzalez-Vergara R, Arroyo-Cazarez JM, Ricardez-Arenas A, del Follo-Valencia A, Padilla-Arriaga S, Veronica Guerrero M, et al. Regression of HPV intraepithelial lesions is induced by MVA E2 therapeutic vaccine. Human Gene Therapy. 2014;**25**:1035-1049. DOI: 10.1089/hum.2014.024

[122] Remy-Ziller C, Germain C, Spindler A, Hoffmann C, Silvestre N, Rooke R, Bonnefoy JY, Préville X. Immunological characterization of a modified vaccinia virus ankara vector expressing the Human Papilloma Virus 16 E1 protein. Clinical and Vaccine Immunology. 2014;**21**:147-155. DOI: 10.1128/CVI.00678-13

[123] Nonn M, Schinz M, Zumbach K, Pawlita M, Schneider A, Dürst M, Kaufmann AM. Dendritic cell-based tumor vaccine for cervical cancer I: *In vitro* stimulation with recombinant protein-pulsed dendritic cells induces specific T cells to HPV16 E7 or HPV18 E7. Journal of Cancer Research and Clinical Oncology. 2003;**129**:511-520

[124] Ferrara A, Nonn M, Sehr P, Schreckenberger C, Pawlita M, Dürst M, Schneider A, Kaufmann AM. Dendritic cell-based tumor vaccine for cervical cancer II: Results of a clinical pilot study in 15 individual patients. Journal of Cancer Research and Clinical Oncology. 2003;**129**:521-530

[125] Santin AD, Bellone S, Palmieri M, Ravaggi A, Romani C, Tassi R, Roman JJ, Burnett A, Pecorelli S, Cannon MJ. HPV16/18 E7-pulsed dendritic cell vaccination in cervical cancer patients with recurrent disease refractory to standard treatment modalities. Gynecologic Oncology. 2006;**100**:469-478

[126] Santin AD, Bellone S, Palmieri M, Zanolini A, Ravaggi A, Siegel ER, Roman JJ, Pecorelli S, Cannon MJ. Human papillomavirus type 16 and 18 E7-pulsed dendritic cell vaccination of stage IB or IIA cervical cancer patients: A phase I escalating-dose trial. Journal of Virology. 2008;**82**:1968-1979

[127] Yin W, Duluc D, Joo H, Oh S. Dendritic cell targeting vaccine for HPV-associated cancer. Cancer Cell and Microenvironment. 2016;**3**:pii: e1482

Section 3

Adjuvants for Human Vaccines

Chapter 3

Anogenital Warts: New Opportunities for Prevention and Treatment

Andrey Dmitrievich Protasov,
Alexander Victorovich Zhestkov,
Yuriy Vladimirovich Tezikov,
Igor Stanislavovich Lipatov,
Mikhail Petrovich Kostinov and
Natal'ya Evgenievna Lavrent'eva

Additional information is available at the end of the chapter

http://dx.doi.org/10.5772/intechopen.69263

Abstract

The study aims at evaluating the efficacy of combined administration of imiquimod 5% crème and human papillomavirus (HPV) quadrivalent recombinant vaccine in order to achieve a long-term clinical remission in patients with chronic HPV infection manifested in condyloma accuminata (CA) of the anogenital area. The study enrolled 36 subjects aged 26.4 (4.1) years (including 22 men) with one to five condyloma accuminata of the anogenital area. Study participants were vaccinated with human papillomavirus quadrivalent recombinant vaccine using a 0–2–6-month regimen with concomitant administration of imiquimod 5% crème applied three times per week for not more than 16 weeks. Patients were monitored over 2 years. Complete disappearance of condyloma accuminata was observed in 34 out of 36 subjects (94.4%) after 1 year from the start of treatment. Two patients still having condyloma accuminata of the anogenital area after 1 year of combination treatment underwent a successful course of treatment with Solcoderm (one patient for 1 year 3 months and the other for 1 year 4 months), which resulted in complete disappearance of condyloma accuminata. Within 2-year period, no recurrence of condyloma accuminata of the anogenital area has been observed.

Keywords: HPV infection, condyloma accuminata, vaccination, human papillomavirus quadrivalent recombinant vaccine, imiquimod, combined administration

1. Introduction

It is well known that 15–20% of all human neoplasms have a viral cause, that is, they are developed due to so-called oncogenic viruses. The experts of the International Agency for Research on Cancer (IARC) consider the following viruses as human oncogenic viruses:

1. RNA viruses:

- Hepatitis B and C viruses (HBV/HCV) causing hepatocellular carcinoma;
- Human T-cell leukemia virus (HTLV-1) which is the etiological agent of adult T-cell leukemia, as well as of tropical spastic paraparesis and several other non-oncologic diseases;
- Human immunodeficiency virus (HIV) which contains no transforming genes yet provides the requisite conditions (immunodeficiency) for the development of cancer.

2. DNA viruses:

- Epstein-Barr virus (EBV) participating in the development of a whole host of malignant tumors, such as Burkitt lymphoma, nasopharyngeal carcinoma, and Hodgkin's lymphoma;
- Human herpesvirus type 8 (HHV-8) playing an important role in the occurrence of Kaposi's sarcoma, primary effusion lymphoma, Castleman disease, and some other pathological conditions;
- Human papillomaviruses (HPV) which are an etiological agent of cervical cancer and several other anogenital tumors.

Considering the severity of and unfavorable prognosis in these diseases, as well as their proven viral etiology, the development of prophylactic methods for such viral infections is becoming a topical issue. Currently, vaccines against hepatitis B virus and HPV are already available.

The problem of HPV infection is one of the most topical health issues in the modern world. According to the World Health Organization (WHO), about half a million new cases of cervical cancer are reported annually worldwide, and 240 thousand women are dying from this disease.

In Russia, symptoms of papillomavirus infection are found in 15.0–34.4% of women aged 19 years or older, and among women attending the gynecology clinic for suspected sexually transmitted diseases, the fraction of HPV-infected subjects is reaching 44.9%. The risk for acquiring HPV infection begins from the moment of a sexual debut and continues throughout an individual's life [1].

HPVs are the oncogenic viruses, that is, they can induce tumors, from harmless to fatal forms. The oncogenic effect is due to their ability to impair differentiation and induce proliferation of the skin and mucosal epitheliocytes which manifest in the form of papillomas (warts) of different types and various localization, as well as epithelial dysplasias which can be transformed into invasive (cancerous) tumors.

Skin warts more often occur in children and usually persist for several years causing only cosmetic inconveniences. The genital (or anogenital) warts are a much more serious condition. They are called condyloma accuminata and form a warty growth that in its typical form resembles the cauliflower. Genital warts more often occur on the outer genitals, although they may affect vagina, cervix, or penis. This is one of the most common sexually transmitted infections [2].

Papillomavirus infection affects both women and men; however, owing to hormonal differences, the likelihood of tumor development in men is much lower than in women. Nonetheless, men can be the HPV carriers for a long time and able to transmit the virus to women.

Papillomaviruses are small (55–60 nm in diameter) non-coated viruses. They are represented by cubical capsids containing two proteins—L1 and L2. The L1 is the major capsid protein comprising more than 80% of capsid material to form the blocks (capsomers) from which the capsid is built.

The anti-L1 antibodies possess the virus-neutralizing activity which underscores the significance of L1 in the initiation of infection. L2 is a minor protein that is not a part of the capsid structure but is involved in capsid stabilization and its coupling with viral genome [3].

Anogenital warts are manifestations of mostly sexually transmitted HPV infection caused by low-oncogenic risk HPV types, such as HPV types 6 and 11. The HPV infections tend to self-resolve on their own but more often they are characterized by recurrent course due to virus persistence. Among the general population, the overall prevalence of HPV infection reaches 80%.

On exceptionally rare occasions, anogenital warts can become cancerous. Anogenital warts may negatively impact patients' quality of life owing to the development of depression and occurrence of psychological and sexual problems [4].

There are numerous approaches for the treatment of anogenital warts (liquid nitrogen cryotherapy, surgical removal, laser therapy, electrocoagulation, use of podophyllotoxin, interferons, imiquimod, and other immune preparations). However, none of the above proved to be ideal. Current therapy for anogenital warts is essentially symptomatic and is aimed at reducing the intensity of symptoms. According to numerous data, the risk of wart recurrence following any type of treatment reaches 30% [4].

One of the new frontiers for solving this problem is the use of an immune preparation imiquimod in combination with HPV quadrivalent recombinant vaccine aiming at eliciting immunity to HPV types 6, 11, 16, and 18. The likely mechanism of combined action of imiquimod and HPV quadrivalent recombinant vaccine is as follows: imiquimod plays an important role in HPV elimination from the infected tissue, while the vaccination using quadrivalent recombinant vaccine promotes specific immune response to prevent re-infection. However, this hypothesis needs to be elaborated and confirmed in further studies using laboratory investigations capable of detecting HPV.

Currently, the following HPV vaccine dosing schedules are being used:

1. A classic three-dose vaccination schedule: 0–2–6 months (i/m in deltoid muscle of arm).

2. An alternative two-dose vaccination schedule: two doses 6 months apart.
3. Three-dose extended schedule: three doses of which the first two are administered within 6 months followed by a booster (third) dose given 5 years later.

Along with the bivalent (Cervarix®) and quadrivalent (Gardasil®) HPV vaccines, currently a 9-valent HPV vaccine (Gardasil-9) has been registered worldwide, which evokes immune response against the following HPV types: 6, 11, 16, 18, 31, 33, 45, 52, and 58. To date, Gardasil-9 is not registered in Russian Federation [5].

The aim of this study is to evaluate the effectiveness of combined use of 5% imiquimod crème and human HPV quadrivalent recombinant vaccine to achieve a durable clinical remission of chronic HPV infection manifesting in anogenital warts.

2. Material and methods

2.1. Clinical characteristics of patients

A single-center, non-randomized, open-label, prospective, pilot study was conducted on 36 patients of whom 22 were men aged 26.4 (4.1) years having from one to five anogenital warts. Among study participants, there were six HIV-infected female patients who received a highly active antiretroviral therapy (four patients received lamivudine 300 mg + abacavir 600 mg + atazanavir 300 mg/ritonavir 100 mg once daily and two patients received lamivudine 300 mg + efavirenz 600 mg once daily plus zidovudine 300 mg twice daily). All six HIV-infected female patients had an undetectable viral load (<50 HIV RNA copies) and CD4+ count >500 cells per 1 μL of blood. The HIV-infected patients represented a population for which the likelihood of immune response to vaccine antigens is ambiguous owing to the presence of possible immune deficiency. We included these patients in the study as at the time of enrollment they had no obvious immune deficiency against a background of highly active antiretroviral therapy. All patients signed the informed consent form.

2.2. Diagnosis of genital warts

The diagnosis of anogenital warts was based on medical history of disease (patients admitted to having unprotected sexual contacts, physician diagnosed the presence of anogenital warts in patient's permanent sex partner) and clinical examination data. Patients with an unequivocal diagnosis, pearly penile papules, or vestibular (labial) papillomatosis were excluded from the study.

Inclusion criteria for the study were as follows:

- Men and women above 18 years of age.
- Presence of one to five anogenital warts.
- Patients with no prior vaccination with human HPV quadrivalent recombinant vaccine.

- Availability of signed and dated informed consent for participation in a pilot study.
- Ability to adhere to study protocol requirements.
- For women of childbearing age—negative pregnancy test before vaccination (the human chorionic gonadotropin test).

Exclusion criteria for the study were as follows:

- Persons under 18 years of age.
- Presence of more than five anogenital warts.
- History of vaccination with human HPV quadrivalent recombinant vaccine.
- Administration of immunoglobulin preparations or blood transfusion within the last 3 months before study commencement.
- Long-term (more than 14 days) use of immunosuppressive drugs within 6 months before study commencement.
- Any confirmed or suspected immunosuppressive or immunodeficiency disorder.
- Respiratory or cardiovascular insufficiency, hepatic, or renal impairment revealed during physical examination during visit 1.
- Marked congenital disorders or exacerbations of serious chronic diseases including any clinically significant exacerbations of chronic pulmonary, liver, kidney, cardiovascular, nervous system, psychiatric diseases, or metabolic disorders confirmed by medical history data or objective examination data.
- History of severe allergic reactions and autoimmune diseases.
- Acute infectious and/or non-infectious diseases within 1 month prior to study commencement.
- Chronic alcohol abuse and/or history of substance abuse.
- Breastfeeding.
- Pregnancy.
- Participation in the other clinical study within the last 3 months.
- Evidence of past or present oncohematologic and other oncologic diseases.

2.3. Intervention

Study participants were prescribed 5% imiquimod crème (Aldara, "MEDA," Sweden) to apply to the warts three times per week before going to sleep followed by washing the cream off with water and soap in the morning. Treatment should last until visible disappearance of anogenital warts but not longer than 16 weeks, and accompanied by concomitant three-dose injection of HPV quadrivalent recombinant vaccine intramuscularly in the deltoid muscle of arm or in the upper outer triceps area using a three-dose series (0–2–6-month schedule). The vaccine is intended for prevention of diseases caused by HPV types 6, 11, 16, and 18, and contains the L1 proteins of the above HPV types. Control visits were made in 1 and 2 years after vaccination. When necessary, patients had an opportunity to contact physician-investigator at any time. According to recent data, vaccination with HPV quadrivalent recombinant vaccine can be done using the "eased" two-shot 0–6-month schedule; however in our study, we used standard 0–2–6-month schedule.

2.4. Safety evaluation

In order to evaluate treatment safety, we collected information about treatment-related adverse events. *Safety of vaccination* was assessed in the following way: after injection of each dose for 7 days, all patients filled in a specially designed questionnaire which included both local and general adverse events. The recorded local adverse events included pain at the injection site (yes/no) and size of a hyperemic focus (in cm). Within a week following vaccination, we also evaluated general (systemic) symptoms, such as body temperature, headache, general malaise, and joint or muscle pain.

Safety of topical application of 5% imiquimod creme was evaluated by the presence of tenderness at the site of crème application and occurrence of ulceration. The information was collected at 6 months after treatment commencement at the time of injection of the third vaccine dose.

2.5. Statistical analysis

Statistical analysis was carried out using the applied software package StatPlus 2009 Professional 5.8.4. The choice of measures of central tendency and measures of dispersion was made based on the type of distribution of variables. The description of quantitative variables corresponding to normal distribution was performed using the mean values (standard deviation) and variables that differ from normally distributed variables as the median values (interquartile range). The qualitative variables were expressed as proportions (%) of the absolute numbers. Also, the 95% confidence intervals were calculated.

3. Results and discussion

3.1. Assessment of safety

3.1.1. First dose

Table 1 shows adverse events for the first 7 days after administration of the first dose of the human papillomavirus quadrivalent recombinant vaccine.

3.1.2. Second dose

Table 2 shows adverse events for the first 7 days after administration of the second dose of the human papillomavirus quadrivalent recombinant vaccine.

Symptoms	1 day	2 day	3 day	4 day	5 day	6 day	7 day	8 day
Pain at the site of injection	30.6 (11/36)	72.2 (26/36)	66.7 (24/36)	61.1 (22/36)	44.4 (16/36)	25 (9/36)	8.3 (3/36)	2.8 (1/36)
Hyperemia at the site of injection of up to 5 cm in size	0 (0/36)	2.8 (1/36)	16.7 (6/36)	22.2 (8/36)	19.4 (7/36)	13.9 (5/36)	5.6 (2/36)	0 (0/36)
Temperature up to 37.5°C	5.6 (2/36)	19.4 (7/36)	5.6 (2/36)	0 (0/36)	0 (0/36)	0 (0/36)	0 (0/36)	0 (0/36)
General malaise	8.3 (3/36)	8.3 (3/36)	30.6 (11/36)	41.7 (15/36)	38.9 (14/36)	25 (9/36)	5.6 (2/36)	2.8 (1/36)
Headache	11.1 (4/36)	27.8 (10/36)	36.1 (13/36)	27.8 (10/36)	33.3 (12/36)	22.2 (8/36)	13.9 (5/36)	16.7 (6/36)
Joint pain or muscle pain	11.1 (4/36)	25 (9/36)	36.1 (13/36)	58.3 (21/36)	50 (18/36)	19.4 (7/36)	13.9 (5/36)	5.6 (2/36)

Table 1. Adverse events for the first 7 days after administration the first dose of the human papillomavirus quadrivalent recombinant vaccine.

Symptoms	1 day	2 day	3 day	4 day	5 day	6 day	7 day	8 day
Pain at the site of injection	22.2 (8/36)	55.6 (20/36)	50 (18/36)	41.7 (15/36)	27.8 (10/36)	22.2 (8/36)	22.2 (8/36)	5.6 (2/36)
Hyperemia at the site of injection of up to 5 cm in size	0 (0/36)	2.8 (1/36)	11.1 (4/36)	5.6 (2/36)	2.8 (1/36)	0 (0/36)	0 (0/36)	0 (0/36)
Temperature up to 37.5°C	2.8 (1/36)	8.3 (3/36)	0 (0/36)	0 (0/36)	0 (0/36)	0 (0/36)	0 (0/36)	0 (0/36)
General malaise	19.4 (7/36)	30.6 (11/36)	19.4 (7/36)	8.3 (3/36)	5.6 (2/36)	0 (0/36)	0 (0/36)	2.8 (1/36)
Headache	11.1 (4/36)	22.2 (8/36)	25 (9/36)	22.2 (8/36)	25 (9/36)	22.2 (8/36)	11.1 (4/36)	13.9 (5/36)
Joint pain or muscle pain	8.3 (3/36)	22.2 (8/36)	38.9 (14/36)	19.4 (7/36)	13.8 (5/36)	5.6 (2/36)	8.3 (3/36)	5.6 (2/36)

Table 2. Adverse events for the first 7 days after administration the second dose of the human papillomavirus quadrivalent recombinant vaccine.

3.1.3. *Third dose*

Table 3 shows adverse events for the first 7 days after administration of the third dose of the human papillomavirus quadrivalent recombinant vaccine.

All vaccination-related adverse events were self-resolved on their own within the first 7 days post-vaccination and required no medication therapy.

Symptoms	1 day	2 day	3 day	4 day	5 day	6 day	7 day	8 day
Pain at the site of injection	13.9 (5/36)	33.3 (12/36)	13.9 (5/36)	2.8 (1/36)	0 (0/36)	0 (0/36)	0 (0/36)	0 (0/36)
Hyperemia at the site of injection of up to 5 cm in size	0 (0/36)	11.1 (4/36)	13.9 (5/36)	5.6 (2/36)	0 (0/36)	0 (0/36)	0 (0/36)	0 (0/36)
Temperature up to 37.5°C	2.8 (1/36)	11.1 (4/36)	0 (0/36)	0 (0/36)	0 (0/36)	0 (0/36)	0 (0/36)	0 (0/36)
General malaise	22.2 (8/36)	36.1 (13/36)	19.4 (7/36)	0 (0/36)	0 (0/36)	0 (0/36)	0 (0/36)	2.8 (1/36)
Headache	13.9 (5/36)	27.8 (10/36)	25 (9/36)	8.3 (5/36)	0 (0/36)	2.7 (1/36)	11.1 (4/36)	0 (0/36)
Joint pain or muscle pain	5.6 (2/36)	27.8 (10/36)	33.3 (12/36)	19.4 (7/36)	11.1 (4/36)	5.6 (2/36)	0 (0/36)	0 (0/36)

Table 3. Adverse events for the first 7 days after administration the third dose of the human papillomavirus quadrivalent recombinant vaccine.

3.2. Assessment of topical administration of 5% imiquimod crème

At 6 months after treatment commencement, all patients reported tenderness at the site of crème application and occurrence of ulcerations which self-resolved on their own in 100% of cases within 14 days after discontinuation of treatment.

All patients completed the study in accordance with study protocol. Patient compliance with treatment was 100%.

3.3. Clinical assessment

At 12 months from study commencement, a complete disappearance of anogenital warts was observed in 34 (94.4%) out of 36 study participants including HIV-infected patients (**Table 4**).

In two patients without HIV infection, the number of anogenital warts decreased from five at baseline to one after 1 year. Two patients with anogenital warts after 1 year, at 1 year 3 months,

Anogenital wart number	At baseline		In 6 months		In 1 year	
	Abs.	%	Abs.	%	Abs.	%
1	4	11.1	2	5.6	2	5.6
2	8	22.2	2	5.6	0	0
3	6	16.7	0	0	0	0
4	4	11.1	0	0	0	0
5	14	38.9	0	0	0	0
Total	36	100	4	11.1	2	5.6

Table 4. Distribution of study participants and observation dynamics in relation to the anogenital wart number.

and 1 year 4 months successfully underwent the treatment course with "Solcoderm," which resulted in complete disappearance of warts. Over the study period, no recurrence of anogenital warts has been found.

Using a given treatment regimen, no clinically significant local or general reactions have been observed.

We have conducted the calculation of several statistical parameters, the results of which are presented in **Table 5**.

The problem to be discussed is not new. However, in author's opinion, a new concept in the treatment of anogenital warts presented in this study deserves attention.

Many authors have been involved in the development of methods of treatment of anogenital warts. Thus, for example, Gomberg and Solovyov [6] reported the use of destructive methods of treatment of anogenital warts, such as electrosurgery, cryosurgery, laser treatment, surgical excision, and laser photothermolysis. It was found that the recurrence rate of anogenital warts does not depend on the selected method of destructive treatment at that. The advantage of these methods is that warts are destroyed quickly and often in a single step. The drawbacks of these methods include the pain caused by the procedure, wart recurrences, requirements in special facility, expensive equipment, and trained medical staff qualified to perform this type of medical activity [6].

Kuznetsova [7] studied the results of treatment of anogenital warts using the application of "Solcoderm" via the capillary tubing with its subsequent mechanical rubbing using a spatula to ensure deeper penetration of the solution. The effectiveness of this method was 80.1%, with the wart recurrence rate of 6–10% within a year. The benefits of this method include treatment

Parameter (formula)	At baseline	In 1 year
Number of patients with AGW	36	2
Chance of AGW presence (n of patients with AGW/n of patients without AGW)	–	2/36 = 0.06
AR (n of patients with AGW/n of patients with AGW risk)	36/36 = 1 = 100%	2/36 = 0.06 = 6%
RR (AR with intervention/AR without intervention), 95% CI	0.06/1 = 0.06 = 6%(0.06; 0.07)*	
ARR (AR with intervention − AR without intervention), 95% CI	0.06 − 1 = −0.94 = −94%(−1.02, −0.86)*	
RRR (difference AR/AR without intervention)	(100% − 6%)/100% = 0.94 = 94%	
NTT (1/ARI)	1/0.94 = 1.06	

AGW, anogenital warts; AR, absolute risk; RR, relative risk; ARR, absolute risk reduction; RRR, relative risk reduction; NTT, number of patients needed to be treated to prevent one unfavorable outcome.

* $P < 0.05$.

Table 5. Statistical parameters (chance, AR, RR, ARR, RRR, and NNT) for study participants over 1 year.

in the outpatient setting, no need for using expensive equipment and anesthesia, absence of scars after treatment, and affordability of treatment. The drawbacks of this method are the recurrence of anogenital warts and the requirement to perform the procedure by a physician.

Apolikhina and Salekh [8] studied the use of podophyllotoxin applied twice daily for 3 days with a subsequent 4-day intermission (duration of treatment did not exceed 5 weeks). The effectiveness of treatment was 87% in men and 77% in women, with the wart recurrence rate of 6–100% within a year. The benefits of podophyllotoxin therapy for anogenital warts included treatment in the outpatient setting, plus the possibility to perform the procedure by a patient without assistance. The drawbacks of this method are wart recurrence, high cost of podophyllotoxin, and long duration of treatment against its not very high effectiveness [8].

Nejmark et al. [9] studied the results of treatment of anogenital warts using isoprinosine which was administered at 3 g/day (two tablets 3 times a day) as an adjunct to topical therapy or surgery for 14–28 days or 5 days a week sequentially for 1–2 weeks per month for 3 months. The effectiveness of combination therapy with isoprinosine was 41–87.5%, and the wart recurrence rate was 7–28%.

The major shortcoming of the above approaches to treatment of anogenital warts is a high wart recurrence rate. In our study, we offer a new approach to solving this problem. The combined use of HPV quadrivalent recombinant vaccine and 5% imiquimod crème aims, on the one hand, at clinical cure (i.e., disappearance of anogenital warts) with possible elimination of the virus, and on the other, at preventing the re-infection with HPV types causing warts with a subsequent long-term remission.

Imiquimod has no direct anti-viral action. Its effect is due to activation of non-specific defense mechanisms and stimulation of TLR7 receptors, induction of synthesis of interferon-alpha and other cytokines which attract to the site of imiquimod application the immunocompetent cells with cytotoxic activity to mediate the anti-viral effect and destroy the virus-infected cells [10–13].

This is a crucial point setting this treatment apart from other therapeutic approaches. Use of imiquimod results not only in visible disappearance of anogenital warts but, perhaps, in the destruction of virus-infected cells that never occurs when other known therapeutic approaches are used. However, this hypothesis needs further exploration as we did not perform laboratory tests for HPV detection.

Imiquimod therapy may lead to clinical remission owing to virus elimination. However, following the imiquimod monotherapy, we observed recurrence of anogenital warts. Perhaps, this is due to incomplete destruction of virus-infected cells, for instance, in immunodeficient patients (e.g., absolute deficit of cytotoxic cells or their functional incompetence), low adherence to imiquimod therapy, or re-infection with HPV type 6 or 11. Overall, the efficacy of annual imiquimod monotherapy varies between 35 and 68%, and the wart recurrence rate between 6 and 26% [14–16].

This pilot study has a number of limitations such as small sampling size, absence of control group, and absence of randomization and placebo control. The well-designed, randomized, placebo-controlled, double-blind, multicenter, prospective studies are needed to elaborate on and confirm our revealed therapeutic effect of combined use of HPV quadrivalent recombinant vaccine and 5% imiquimod crème in the treatment of anogenital warts to achieve a long-term clinical remission. The issue of virologic cure using this therapeutic approach also awaits clarification.

Our developed approach to the treatment of anogenital warts using the HPV quadrivalent recombinant vaccine and 5% imiquimod crème demonstrated high clinical effectiveness. However, in designing future clinical studies on this subject, a special attention should be paid to laboratory investigation of HPV DNA carrier state in studied patient population to verify our hypothesis on the virologic cure. Nonetheless, our data are important as they provide a new insight into the possibility of complete HPV elimination in a given patient cohort [11, 12].

4. Conclusions

Vaccination with HPV quadrivalent recombinant vaccine using a three-dose vaccination schedule (0–2–6 months) and a concurrent 5% imiquimod crème application three times daily for not more than 16 weeks ensures the achievement of a long-term clinical remission of chronic HPV infection which is manifested in anogenital warts in at least 94.4% of cases over a 2-year follow-up. This treatment method proved to be safe. The adverse events observed during combined vaccination and 5% imiquimod crème administration were, as a rule, mild and self-resolved on their own (within 7 days following vaccination and within 14 days after discontinuation of 5% imiquimod crème). Clinical significance of these results awaits confirmation in future studies supported by methods of laboratory diagnosis.

Author details

Andrey Dmitrievich Protasov[1]*, Alexander Victorovich Zhestkov[1], Yuriy Vladimirovich Tezikov[1], Igor Stanislavovich Lipatov[1], Mikhail Petrovich Kostinov[2] and Natal'ya Evgenievna Lavrent'eva[1]

*Address all correspondence to: crosss82@mail.ru

1 Samara State Medical University, Samara, Russian Federation

2 Mechnikov Research Institute of Vaccines and Sera, Moscow, Russian Federation

References

[1] Mayanskii AN. Human papilloma virus—Oncogenic virus. Pediatric Pharmacology. 2010; **7**(4):48-55 (in Russian)

[2] Stanley M. Immunobiology of HPV and HPV vaccines. Gynecologic Oncology. 2008;**109**(2): S15-S21. DOI: 10.1016/j.ygyno.2008.02.003

[3] Osazuwa-Peters N. Human papillomavirus (HPV), HPV-associated oropharyngeal cancer, and HPV vaccine in the United States—Do we need a broader vaccine policy? Vaccine. 2013;**31**(47):5500-5505. DOI: 10.1016/j.vaccine.2013.09.031

[4] Howell-Jones R, de Silva N, Akpan M, Oakeshott P, Carder C, Coupland L, et al. Prevalence of human papillomavirus (HPV) infections in sexually active adolescents and young women in England, prior to widespread HPV immunization. Vaccine. 2012;**30**(26):3867-3875. DOI: 10.1016/j.vaccine.2012.04.006

[5] Turner TB, Huh WK. HPV vaccines: Translating immunogenicity into efficacy. Human Vaccines and Immunotherapeutics. 2015;**12**(6):1403-1405. DOI: 10.1080/21645515.2015.1103936

[6] Gomberg MA, Solovyov AM. Carbuncle and pointed condyloma treatment—Easy and effective. Medical Council. 2011;**5-6**:60-65 (in Russian)

[7] Kuznetsova YN. Treatment of genital warts with solkoderm. Urals Medical Journal. 2005;**3**:2-3 (in Russian)

[8] Apolikhina IA, Salekh YV. Current possibilities in the treatment of pointed condylomas. Obstetrics and Gynecology. 2011;**5**:134-136 (in Russian)

[9] Nejmark BA, Kondrat'eva YS, Zologina VS, Torbik DV. Effectiveness of combined treatment of HPV infection. Urology. 2015;**2**:39-42 (in Russian)

[10] Hengge UR, Benninghoff B, Ruzicka T, Goos M. Topical immunomodulators—Progress towards treating inflammation, infection, and cancer. The Lancet Infectious Diseases. 2001;**1**(3):189-198. DOI: 10.1016/s1473-3099(01)00095-0

[11] Gaspari AA, Sauder DN. Immunotherapy of basal cell carcinoma: Evolving approaches. Dermatologic Surgery. 2003;**29**(10):1027-1034. DOI: 10.1046/j.1524-4725.2003.29295.x

[12] Stanley MA. Imiquimod and the imidazoquinolones: Mechanism of action and therapeutic potential. Clinical and Experimental Dermatology. 2002;**27**(7):571-577. DOI: 10.1046/j.1365-2230.2002.01151.x

[13] Sauder DN. Immunomodulatory and pharmacologic properties of imiquimod. Journal of the American Academy of Dermatology. 2000;**43**(1):S6-S11. DOI: 10.1067/mjd.2000.107808

[14] Protasov AD, Lipatov IS, Kostinov MP, Tezikov YV, Shmitko AD, Pakhomov DV, Blagovidov DA, Zhestkov AV, Ryzhov AA, Vekhova EV. Anogenital warts: A new way of solving the common problem of urology (results of long-term follow-up). Urology. 2016;**5**:47-51 (in Russian)

[15] Jurk M, Heil F, Vollmer J, Schetter C, Krieg AM, Wagner H, Lipford G, Bauer S. Human TLR7 or TLR8 independently confer responsiveness to the antiviral compound R-848. Nature Immunology. 2002;**3**(6):499. DOI: 10.1038/ni0602-499

[16] Protasov AD, Tezikov YV, Kostinov MP, Lipatov IS, Magarshak OO, Ryzhov AA. Combined use of vaccination and immunotherapy drugs to achieve a long-term clinical remission in patients with chronic HPV-infection manifested in condyloma accuminata of the anogenital area. Epidemiology and Vaccinal Prevention. 2016;**3**(88):60-66 (in Russian)

Chapter 4

The Efficacy of Immunoadjuvant-Containing Influenza Vaccines in Pregnancy

Kostinov Mikhail Petrovich,
Cherdantsev Alexander Petrovich,
Shmitko Anna Dmitrievna,
Akhmatova Nelly Kimovna,
Kostinova Aristitsa Mikhailovna,
Praulova Darya Alexandrovna,
Polyschuk Valentina Borisovna,
Protasov Andrey Dmitrievich,
Zhestkov Alexander Victorovich and
Tezikov Yuriy Vladimirovich

Additional information is available at the end of the chapter

http://dx.doi.org/10.5772/intechopen.69271

Abstract

The aim of the work was to determine the clinical safety and immunogenicity of immunoadjuvant vaccines against influenza (MonoGripol Plus and Grippol® Plus) in 182 pregnant women in the II and III trimesters of gestation , and further assessment of fetal conditions and infants of the first 6 months of life. Results: It was shown that immunoadjuvant vaccines do not have a negative effect on the physiological course of pregnancy and the functional state of the fetoplacental complex. In the early postpartum period, the rates of physical and neuro-psychological development and the nature of feeding of children did not differ from the control group. In pregnant women vaccinated with Grippol® plus, the levels of seroprotection to strains of A/H1N1/v are 82.0%, A/H3N2/—88.0%, B—88.3% that measure the CPMP criteria and last more than a year . After birth, transplacental antibodies in children in protective values were observed in 52.3–68.9% of cases, did not differ from the control group, and disappear after 6 months. Respiratory infections during the first 6 months of life of infants born from mothers vaccinated against influenza registered in 1.8 times less frequently.

Keywords: pregnant women, vaccine against influenza, post-vaccination immunity.

1. Introduction

The reports of Strategic Advisory Group of Experts (SAGE) on Immunization underscore that between 7 and 10% of all hospitalized patients with severe influenza are women in the second and third trimester of pregnancy. The requirements of pregnant women with influenza infection for providing medical care in an intensive care unit are 10 times that of other population groups diagnosed with influenza [1–4].

Vaccination of pregnant women using the subunit and split influenza vaccines is routinely performed in a number of countries of Europe and America for over 20 years, and the vaccine efficacy reaches 70–85% [5, 6]. Clinical studies have shown that vaccination of pregnant women using modern inactivated influenza vaccines neither affect the course of pregnancy and fetal growth nor cause undesirable post-vaccination effects. It was found that vaccination of pregnant women using inactivated influenza vaccines leads to 50–63% reduction of flu-related morbidity among infants up to 6 months of age [7, 8].

The WHO Global Advisory Committee on Vaccine Safety indicates that influenza vaccination is a non-alternative approach to safe and effective prevention of influenza in pregnancy [1, 9, 10]. In Russia, the indications for vaccination of pregnant women using modern vaccines are defined within the National Immunization Program Schedule of Russian Federation (RF) (order of Ministry of Healthcare of Russian Federation №125n of 21 March 2014). Federal clinical guidelines "Influenza vaccination of pregnant women" and manuals for physicians have been published which establish the main vaccination requirements for the primary health care in Russia [11–13].

The unfavorable epidemiological situation with influenza that occurred in 2009 has accelerated the development and implementation in healthcare practices of adjuvant-containing pandemic influenza vaccines such as Fluad (containing squalene) and Arepanrix™H1N1 (containing AS03—squalene + α-Tocopherol acetate) which confer enhanced immunogenicity [1, 14]. Adjuvants accelerate, change the dynamics of development of the immunity, and increase its level and the duration of persistence of post-vaccination antibodies. With the help of an adjuvant, durable and solid immunity is achieved by administering small doses of antigen and a less number of injections.

In Russia, two adjuvant-containing subunit influenza vaccines have been developed (monovalent (pandemic) and trivalent preparations). These drugs, in contrast to non-adjuvant subunit vaccines against influenza (e.g., Agrippal S1 containing 15 μg strains of influenza viruses type A and B), have 5 μg of both strains of the influenza virus and an adjuvant-immunomodulator polyoxidonium. In clinical trials, immunoadjuvant vaccines demonstrated high efficacy and safety in children aged 6 months and older and in adults. The trivalent adjuvant-based influenza vaccine is used in clinical practice for more than 20 years [15–24]. In experimental studies, these vaccines showed no teratogenic effect on the developing fetus. Despite extensive use of these vaccines for specific prevention of influenza in Russia, studies on their safety in pregnancy have not been conducted until recently. The information on the effects of adjuvant-containing vaccines on the fetus and post-natal development was missing. The information on vaccine immunogenicity for pregnant women at different gestational age, as well as vaccine ability to confer an adequate passive immunity to a fetus, was insufficient.

The study aimed at determining clinical safety and immunogenicity of "MonoGrippol Plus" and "Grippol® Plus" vaccines in pregnant women in the second and third trimesters of pregnancy with assessment of fetal condition and condition of infants during the first 6 months of life.

2. Materials and methods

2.1. Legal basis of the research

The study was carried out according to the protocol which met the National standard of Russian Federation—GOST P 52379-2005 "Good Clinical Practice" and the international GCP (good clinical practice) standards. Vaccination of pregnant women was carried out with adherence to the ethical norms and guidelines of the WHO and Ministry of Health care of RF.

Women to be vaccinated and followed up were selected strictly in accordance with a case report form that was examined and approved by the Ethics Committee of the Ulyanovsk State University (protocol №35 of 14.01.2010).

The observation of pregnant women before and after vaccination was carried out jointly with an obstetrician-gynecologist in accordance with requirements of the Order of Ministry of Health care and Social Development of RF of 02.10.2009 N 808n "On the approval of the Order of providing obstetric and gynecologic care." Before vaccination, women underwent laboratory testing after they have given the informed consent to participate in the study (**Figure 1**).

During observation and examination of infants, we also adhered to the ethical requirements applicable to biomedical studies. Development of the order and scope of studied parameters was based on provisions listed in the Order № 370 of Ministry of Healthcare of RF of 28.04.2007.

2.2. Randomization

The study was a randomized, placebo-controlled, single-blind, comparative, parallel-group study conducted on pregnant women and infants.

All candidates for study program underwent a preliminary assessment of whether they met the protocol inclusion and exclusion criteria (in accordance with the GMP standards).

Eligibility criteria:

1. Healthy pregnant women aged 20–40.
2. Volunteers capable of fulfilling the protocol requirements (i.e., able to fill in the self-observation diary and turn up for the scheduled visits).
3. Written informed consent of the volunteers to participate in the clinical study.

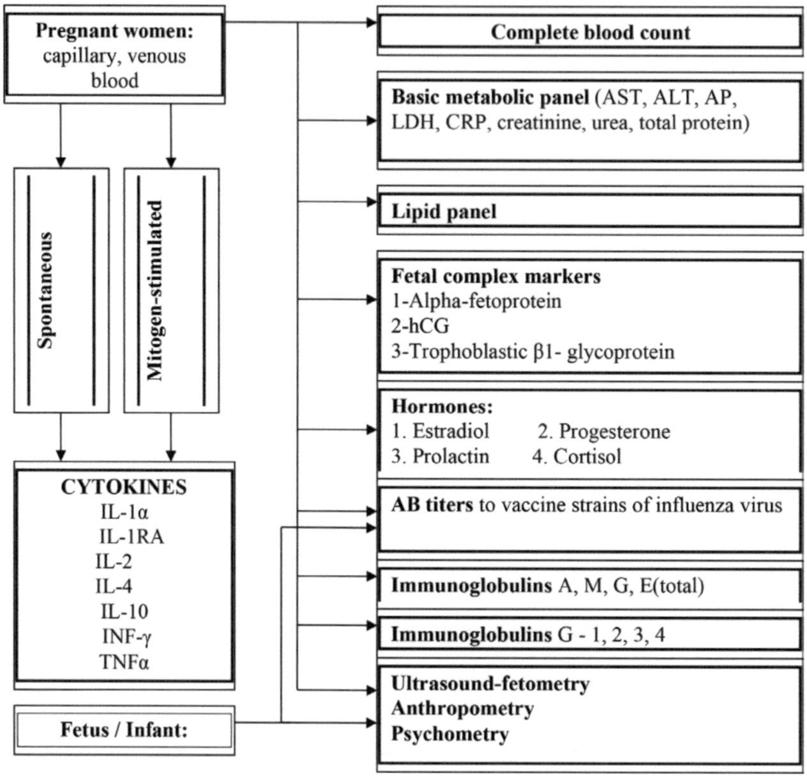

Figure 1. An algorithm of laboratory, physical and instrumental investigation.

Exclusion criteria:

1. History of leukemia, oncologic conditions or positive tests for HIV, hepatitis B and C.
2. Volunteers who had received the immunoglobulin preparations or blood transfusions within the last three months prior to the study.
3. Long-term (more than 14 days) administration of immunodepressants or other immunomodulating drugs within the last six months prior to the study.
4. Any confirmed or suspected immunosuppressive or immunodeficiency disorder.
5. History of chronic alcohol abuse and/or substance abuse.
6. Presence of respiratory or cardiovascular insufficiency, hepatic or renal impairment revealed during physical examination or by laboratory tests at visit 1.
7. Severe congenital defects or serious chronic diseases including any clinically significant diseases of lungs, kidneys, cardiovascular system, nervous system, psychiatric diseases or metabolic disorders confirmed by anamnestic data or objective clinical examination.

8. Presence of acute infectious and/or non-infectious diseases at the time of enrollment in the study.

9. Pregnancy via IVF procedure.

2.3. Duration of observation

A total number of pregnant women vaccinated against influenza during the epidemic seasons of 2009–2010, 2010–2011, and 2011–2012 were 345 subjects. Of those, the number of women and their children participated in an in-depth examination and their assignment to groups and subgroups is presented in **Table 1**.

The frequency of clinical examination and blood collection for laboratory testing in the post-vaccination period was based on the gestational age at the start of observation. Women vaccinated in the second and third trimesters underwent 7 and 6 examinations, respectively.

2.4. Assessment of fetal conditions

Fetometric measurements were carried out using the ultrasound (US) examination during pregnancy weeks 21–22 and 33–35 and included determination and calculation of biparietal diameter (BPD), fronto-occipital size (FOS), head circumference (HC), abdominal circumference (AC), estimated fetal weight (FW) and the femur length/abdominal circumference (FL/AC) ratio. The generally accepted guidelines were followed to evaluate the parameters obtained.

2.5. Assessment of infant conditions

Infant observation started from the first hours and days of life (day 2–3) and was conducted jointly with a neonatologist at maternity home. The basic signs of functional and morphological maturity of the newborn (Apgar score), blood work parameters/biochemical profile and antibody levels to influenza virus strains have been analyzed. All newborns at maternity home underwent neurosonography and cardiac sonography. Basic anthropometric measurements included body weight (BW), body length (BL), head circumference (HC), chest circumference (CC), and height-weight index (Ketle 1).

At the age of 3 and 6 months, the main parameters of physical and neuropsychological development and feeding pattern have been recorded.

2.6. Hormonal status in pregnant women

Hormone concentration in pregnant women was measured using the licensed immunoenzyme test-systems (IETS) such as "Estradiol-EIA" (LLC "Chema," Germany), "EIA-Progesterone,"

	Group I Pregnant women vaccinated with "MonoGrippol Plus"		Group II Pregnant women vaccinated with "Grippol® Plus"		Group III Pregnant women vaccinated with "Agrippal S1"		Group IV Pregnant women who had received "Placebo"		Group V Non-pregnant women, who had received	
	Trimesters of pregnancy								MonoGrippol Plus	Grippol Plus
	II	III	II	III	II	III	II	III		
Number of women participated in study program	28	15	27	23	27	21	22	19	30	19
Total:	43		50		48		41		49	
Average age (years)	25.1 ± 0.7		23.3 ± 0.4		27.8 ± 0.6		24.1 ± 0.3		23.1 ± 0.4	
Number of children born to women vaccinated during pregnancy	24	14	27	21	23	19	18	17		
Total:	38		48		42		35			

Table 1. Study participants' assignment to observation groups.

"EIA-Prolactin," "EIA-Cortisol" (LLC "Alcor Bio Company, Russia"). Fetoplacental complex markers, such as serum alpha-fetoprotein (AFP), human chorionic gonadotropin (hCG) and trophoblastic β1-glycoprotein (TBG), were tested using the IETS from CJSC "Vector-Best," Russia.

2.7. Cytokine profile

Serum cytokines were measured to determine levels of interleukin-1α (IL-1α), interleukin-2 (IL-2), interleukin-4 (IL-4), interferon-γ (IFN-γ), tumor necrosis factor α (TNFα), interleukin-1α receptor antagonist (IL-1RA), and interleukin-10 (IL-10). We used a dual cytokine assay to measure spontaneous and mitogen-induced cytokine production using a system of sample preparation from "Cytokine-Stimul-Best" (CJSC "Vector-Best", Russia). As the test systems, we used standard EIA kits (CJSC "Vector-Best" and LLC "Cytokine", Russia).

2.8. Humoral immune response to vaccination

Concentration of serum immunoglobulins A, M, G, E and IgG subclasses was determined using the appropriate IETS from CJSC "Vector-Best," Russia. Titers of antibodies to influenza virus strains A and B were measured in the hemagglutination inhibition test (HAI) as recommended by the WHO for this kind of studies. As viral antigens, we used the A/California/7/2009/H1N1/v-like, A/H3N2/(Victoria)-like and B (Brisbane)-like strains provided by the laboratory of artificial antigens (FSFI "State Research Center at the Institute of Immunology" of FMBA, Russia).

Vaccine immunogenicity was determined based on criteria established by the Committee for Proprietary Medicinal Products (CPMP) according to the protocol CPMP/BWP/214/96:

1. *Seroprotection level* (>70%).
2. *Seroconversion level* or *vaccine immunologic activity* (>40%).
3. *Seroconversion factor* or *geometric mean fold rise* (>2.5).

2.9. Vaccines

All vaccines used in the study were subunit inactivated preparations. Development of "MonoGrippol Plus" and "Grippol® Plus" vaccines (LLC "NPO Petrovax Pharm," Russia) is based on a special technology of coupling of highly purified protective influenza virus antigens with a polymeric, water-soluble, high-molecular weight adjuvant polyoxidonium. This technology enables a threefold reduction of hemagglutinin (HA) of each viral strain (down to 5 μg) in the vaccine compared to the analog subunit, adjuvant-free vaccine "Agrippal S1" ("Novartis Vaccines and Diagnostics," Italy).

"MonoGrippol Plus" contains antigens of only one influenza virus strain, namely A/California/7/2009/H1N1/v and belongs to the monovalent pandemic influenza vaccines, whereas

"Grippol Plus" and "Agrippal S1" additionally contain antigens of other strains, that is, A/H3N2/(Victoria)-like and B/Brisbane-like (trivalent vaccines).

2.10. Placebo

As a placebo, we used phosphate buffer saline ("GlaxoSmithKline Biologicals") which is used as a diluent for lyophilized vaccines.

2.11. Vaccination

Vaccination of pregnant women was performed in the vaccination room with adherence to sanitary and hygiene regulations, with emergency care available at once. Vaccine preparations were injected intramuscularly as a single-dose of 0.5 mL in the upper third of the arm (deltoid muscle).

2.12. Evaluation of vaccination safety

After an injection, the woman was observed for 40 min for the adverse reaction(s), which were scored to categorize reactions as described in **Table 2**.

Local reactions	
0—absent	Absence of symptoms
1—mild	Hyperemia up to 50 mm in diameter or infiltrate up to 25 mm in diameter
2—moderate	Hyperemia over 50 mm in diameter or infiltrate 26–50 mm in diameter
3—severe	Infiltrate over 50 mm in diameter
Systemic reactions	
0—absent	Absence of symptoms
1—mild	Presence of mild symptoms
2—moderate	Symptoms which markedly impair normal daily activity
3—severe	Symptoms which interfere with normal daily activity
Fever	
0—absent	≤37°C
1—mild	>37°C to ≤37.5°C
2—moderate	>37.6°C to ≤38.5°C
3—severe	>38.6°C

Table 2. Assessment of undesirable post-vaccination reactions.

All possible changes in the well-being and health state were recorded in the case report form (CRF) and self-observation diary (SOD) which the women continued to fill in on a daily basis throughout the first month of the follow-up.

2.13. Statistical analysis

Statistical analysis of samples which did not follow a normally distributed pattern was carried out using the non-parametric tools or parametric methods when the samples followed a normal distribution. We used the applied software package "Microsoft Excel" with the "AtteStat" application (version 10.10.2.). The differences were considered significant at $p < 0.05$.

3. Results and discussion

3.1. Particulars of the course of pregnancy in women vaccinated with "Grippol® Plus"

Although many pregnant women had a history of somatic diseases before they entered the study, as a rule, no exacerbation of pre-existing disease has been observed. The most commonly encountered illness was a mild hypochromic anemia (60.5, 70.0, 61.3, and 60.9% of pregnant women in group I–IV, respectively). Markers of chronic urogenital infection were detected fairly often (44.2% in group I, 46.0% in group II, 59.1% in group III, and 41.5% in group IV). Also, the syndrome of vegetative dystonia (20.9% in group I, 38.0% in group II, 20.5% in group III, and 29.3% in group IV) and altered allergic response (16.3% in group I, 20.0% in group II, 18.2% in group III, and 19.5% in group IV) had been observed. All women had approximately the same frequency of cases of threatened miscarriage in the past (53.5% in group I, 48.0% in group II, 47.7% in group III, and 51.2% in group IV). Therefore, clinical condition of pregnant women was comparable among the groups [25].

3.1.1. Clinical course of the post-vaccination period

Evaluation of the clinical course of the post-vaccination period has shown that it was asymptomatic in 58.1% of women from group I, 60.0% from group II, 54.5% from group III, and 60.9% from group IV ($p > 0.05$). It came under notice that in groups I, II, and III, women vaccinated in the third trimester of pregnancy developed the post-vaccination local and systemic undesirable effects significantly less often than women vaccinated in the second trimester ($p < 0.05$ to $p < 0.01$). The local symptoms occurred in the first few days after vaccination included pain, hyperemia, and infiltration at the site of injection. Such reactions occurred more often in pregnant women immunized with trivalent vaccines (group II—8.0%, group III—10.4%) than in women from placebo group (4.9%), ($p < 0.05$). It was noted that pregnant women from group I developed no or minimal systemic adverse reactions (nausea, fatigability, dizziness or myalgia) where intensity was significantly lower compared to that in women vaccinated with trivalent vaccine, namely group I—6.9% ($p < 0.05$ versus group II), group II—12.0%, group III—10.4%, and group IV—10.2% [26, 27].

3.1.2. *Clinical blood analysis*

In the late (8–30 days) post-vaccination period, no local post-injection reactions have been reported in either group. Systemic reactions included frequent complaints on increased fatigability and headaches in women from group III ($p < 0.05$). With regard to other symptoms, the groups did not differ significantly between each other and the placebo group (group I—9.3%, group II—14.0%, group III—12.5%, and group IV—12.2%). All symptoms were of a transient nature and required no medication management [26, 27].

Analysis of complete blood count has shown that for the majority of formed elements, cell counts did not differ from normal values in both pre-vaccination and post-vaccination periods. Occasional differences were mostly related to the particulars of the pregnancy period. Analysis of basic metabolic panel performed in dynamics on day 7 and day 30 of the post-vaccination period in each group also did not reveal significant abnormalities which could reflect changes in the metabolic homeostasis ($p > 0.05$). Small changes in creatinine level (minimal value in group III at day 30 post-vaccination—58.04 ± 1.57 μmol/L) and alkaline phosphatase (AP) (maximum value in group III at day 30 post-vaccination—86.23 ± 7.84 IU/L) are not remarkable and fall within the average normal values, attesting to normal variability of this parameter [28, 29].

3.1.3. *Lipid metabolism*

Analysis of lipid panel obtained 30 days post-vaccination has shown that in all groups, the parameters of lipid/cholesterol metabolism are not significantly altered, and remain within physiological variations [12, 13].

3.1.4. *Hormonal profile*

Analysis of hormonal profile among vaccinated women has revealed only the intra-group changes in hormone levels which are not so much related to vaccination but rather are due to the gestational age.

Significant differences in prolactin, progesterone, estradiol, and cortisol serum levels were observed in women of different gestational age regardless of whether they received monovalent or trivalent influenza vaccine or placebo ($p < 0.05$). Therefore, it can be affirmed that, despite certain differences in the composition of influenza vaccines used in the study, there are no hormonal changes which could have influenced the state of the fetoplacental unit [12, 13].

3.1.5. *Humoral immunity*

Serum levels of immunoglobulins measured immediately after vaccination and on day 7 post-vaccination were comparable in pregnant women immunized with different influenza vaccines. At day 30, post-vaccination pregnant women who had received the monovalent influenza vaccine demonstrated higher IgA levels (2.56 ± 0.27 mg/mL) compared to women vaccinated with trivalent preparations (1.61 ± 0.09 mg/mL in group II, 1.34 ± 0.11 mg/mL in group III, and 1.14 ± 0.14 mg/mL in group IV) ($p < 0.01$ to $p < 0.001$). Despite the above differences, the antibody levels reflect normal serum IgA variations. Despite the established difference, the IgA content in all comparison groups was recorded within the physiological norm. Levels of IgM and IgG antibodies did not differ significantly between the groups.

Some variations in the IgG subclasses (1, 2, 3, 4) in the early and late post-vaccination periods were found. However, these variations remained within the acceptable range. In pregnant women with a history of allergic diseases, vaccination against influenza had no subsequent effect on serum total IgE levels.

3.1.6. Cytokine profile

It was noted that all pregnant women vaccinated with different vaccine preparations had elevated levels of mitogen-stimulated IL-1α at day 7 post-vaccination. By day 30, concentration of IL-1α remained elevated as compared to placebo control ($p < 0.05$) although was significantly lower than in vaccinated non-pregnant women ($p < 0.01$). No changes in the IL-2 and TNFα levels have been observed in vaccinated pregnant women although were also significantly higher than in non-pregnant women ($p < 0.01$). The IL-1RA values in a spontaneous cytokine production assay were significantly elevated only after vaccination with trivalent preparations by day 7 (group II) and by day 30 (groups II and III) post-vaccination ($p < 0.01$). At the same time, following mitogen stimulation, no significant changes in the IL-2 concentration have been found in any group. All pregnant women demonstrated significant increase in the IL-IRA and IL-10 following mitogen stimulation regardless of the type of vaccine that reflected the mechanism of physiological control of immune activation.

The IL-4 levels were most stable, with no significant dynamic changes among the groups. The only exception was a subgroup of women immunized with a non-adjuvanted trivalent vaccine in different trimesters of pregnancy. It was noted that by day 7 post-vaccination, a higher level of stimulated IL-4 was found in vaccinated women in the third trimester of pregnancy (6.85 ± 0.11 pg/mL in group III) as compared to pregnant women who had received the adjuvant-containing vaccine during the same period (2.95 ± 0.09 pg/mL in group II) ($p < 0.05$). Subsequently (on day 30 post-vaccination), such differences between the groups could not be found.

Pregnant women had lower IFNγ levels in the mitogen-stimulated cytokine production assay (881.86 ± 92.93 pg/mL in group I, 784.17 ± 65.03 pg/mL in group II, 854.89 ± 68.71 pg/mL in group III, and 790.30 ± 45.55 pg/mL in group IV) than the non-pregnant women (1419.60 ± 69.45 pg/mL in group V) which reflected a natural background level of physiological immune response ($p < 0.05$). At the same time during the first 7 days, post-vaccination elevated IFNγ was detected only in pregnant women who had received the polymer-subunit vaccines (6.47 ± 1.68 pg/mL in group I and 5.89 ± 1.08 pg/mL in group II) as compared to group III (3.03 ± 0.39 pg/mL) ($p < 0.05$). These differences were short-lived, and by day 30, post-vaccination was undetectable [30].

Therefore, the overall picture of cytokine profile in pregnant women had a trend characteristic of physiologic immunosuppression in pregnancy, that is, moderately elevated IL-IRA and

IL-10 and the absence in the post-vaccination period of significantly elevated anti-inflammatory cytokines in the mitogen-stimulation cytokine production assay. Nonetheless, the adjuvanted subunit vaccines had certain differences in their ability to influence cytokine secretion and short-term elevation of IFNγ which is most prominent in women in the second trimester of pregnancy that may reflect active involvement of the Th_1-mediated mechanisms of post-vaccination immunity. Use of non-adjuvanted vaccines leads to immune processes in the early post-vaccination period which are accompanied by increased IL-4 synthesis by blood leukocytes (a sign of Th_2-mediated activation) especially in women vaccinated in late pregnancy. The indirect evidence in favor of this suggestion is the absence of significance changes in the IFNγ levels in the early and late post-vaccination periods. All found changes of parameters recorded in different groups of vaccinated women remained within an acceptable range of variation. Also, no changes pertaining to destabilization of regulation and functioning of immune system due to influenza vaccination of pregnant women have been found [31].

3.2. Effect of vaccination of pregnant women using "Grippol® Plus" influenza vaccine on the antenatal fetal development

3.2.1. Fetoplacental complex

Monitoring of fetal development was carried out using a complex of measures, which included analysis of markers of fetoplacental complex and ultrasound fetometry. In all groups of women in the early and late post-vaccination period, no changes in the basic parameters of embryo/fetogenesis (AFP, hCG, TBG) have been found (**Table 3**). Changes in the above parameters did not depend on the type of influenza vaccine used and corresponded to the gestational age (second and third trimesters of pregnancy). Thus, for example, the TBG level in all

Parameter		**Group I "MonoGrippol Plus" (n = 43)**	**Group II "Grippol® Plus" (n = 50)**	**Group III "Agrippal S1" (n = 48)**	**Group IV "Placebo" (n = 41)**
In 7 days	TBG Ng/mL	97.93 ± 20.97	72.69 ± 11.89	88.04 ± 15.46	92.69 ± 20.88
	AFP IU/mL	60.05 ± 13.39	69.59 ± 7.62	81.09 ± 17.88	75.41 ± 10.36
	hCG IU/mL	36.51 ± 4.62	39.74 ± 8.22	40.43 ± 3.10	36.15 ± 2.48
In 30 days	TBG Ng/mL	124.85 ± 14.43	109.17 ± 10.81	118.21 ± 13.99	110.35 ± 13.12
	AFP IU/mL	98.65 ± 8.33	100.43 ± 11.01	110.84 ± 11.19	115.29 ± 9.92
	hCG IU/mL	29.52 ± 3.62	33.84 ± 7.55	29.24 ± 5.20	28.95 ± 1.88

Note: $p > 0.05$ for differences between groups.

Table 3. Fetal complex markers in pregnant women vaccinated against influenza (M ± m).

groups (including placebo control) of women vaccinated in the second trimester of pregnancy was significantly lower than in the third trimester ($p < 0.05$ to $p < 0.01$). A direct relationship was found between the TBG and AFP concentrations ($r = 0.60$; $p < 0.05$) with TBG levels rising as pregnancy progresses ($p < 0.001$). The hCG levels were dropping during the follow-up and inversely correlated with the TBG levels ($r = -0.50$; $p < 0.01$). All serum markers had no deviations from the reference values and reflected physiological changes in pregnancy [32].

3.2.2. Fetometry

Fetometry performed in the second (21–22 weeks) and third (33–35 `) trimester of pregnancy failed to reveal differences among the groups of pregnant women (**Table 4**).

Therefore, study results indicate that vaccination of pregnant women using the adjuvant-containing influenza vaccines "MonoGrippol Plus" and "Grippol® Plus" has no effect on the intrauterine fetal development. Changes of the basic parameters of fetoplacental unit are comparable between the groups and reflect physiological changes during fetal growth.

3.3. Pregnancy outcomes in women vaccinated with "MonoGrippol Plus" and "Grippol® Plus" influenza vaccines

In the majority of cases (85.4–90.7%), pregnancy resulted in physiologic birth (**Table 5**). In a fraction of women, their pregnancy terminated prematurely with the birth of preterm babies (between 2.0 and 8.3%) which corresponds to the preterm birth rate in the Ulyanovsk region of Russia (3.7–5.8%) where the study was taking place. Such outcome was due to the obstetric pathology which was unrelated to prior vaccination. Also, cases of birth of babies with perinatally acquired neurological impairment were mostly associated with gestational immaturity (7.3–10.4%). A fraction of babies had the intrauterine infection-like syndrome (2.0–6.3%) and developmental abnormalities and defects in 2.0–4.9% of cases (3.8–5.9% across the Ulyanovsk region) [33]. Owing to the above abnormalities, such babies were excluded from further study.

3.4. Particulars of development of up to 6 month old infants born to mothers vaccinated during pregnancy with "MonoGrippol Plus" and "Grippol® Plus" influenza vaccines

3.4.1. Apgar scale

The early neonatal period of infants born to mothers vaccinated during pregnancy had a comparable dynamics between the groups. It was shown that, immediately after birth, the number of babies with Apgar score of 8–9 points was similar between the groups (group I—92.1%, group II—87.5%, group III—80.9%, and group IV—94.3%) which attests to the overall good functional maturity. The period of adaptation in newborns passed without complications [34, 35].

3.4.2. Feeding

The feeding of infants born to mothers vaccinated with different influenza vaccines did not differ significantly between the groups. The highest number of nursing mothers (100%) during the neonatal period was observed in groups I and IV and was somewhat lower in groups

Clinical groups	Gestational age	Parameter					
		BPD (mm)	FOS (mm)	HC (mm)	AC (mm)	Fetal weight (g)	$\frac{FL}{AC} \times 100$ (%)
Group I "MonoGrippol Plus" (n = 43)	21–22 weeks	53.18 ± 3.20	73.87 ± 8.11	188.12 ± 13.72	162.81 ± 17.08	527.10 ± 92.31	21.54 ± 0.57
	33–35 weeks	87.81 ± 5.52	111.67 ± 12.9	313.01 ± 24.18	311.60 ± 18.57	2539.40 ± 437.10	22.04 ± 0.44
Group II "Grippol® Plus" (n = 50)	21–22 weeks	54.04 ± 2.70	70.07 ± 7.42	183.90 ± 11.86	170.11 ± 15.98	504.70 ± 96.01	19.49 ± 0.86
	33–35 weeks	89.11 ± 5.31	109.80 ± 14.20	304.21 ± 38.73	295.90 ± 21.07	2489.70 ± 367.30	23.13 ± 0.78
Group III "Agrippal S1" (n = 48)	21–22 weeks	52.56 ± 2.62	68.55 ± 8.12	180.87 ± 18.66	175.44 ± 16.08	489.50 ± 110.10	20.26 ± 0.93
	33–35 weeks	81.49 ± 6.53	106.12 ± 11.40	301.01 ± 21.74	298.30 ± 33.15	2595.2 ± 455.1	22.96 ± 1.04
Group IV "Placebo" (n = 41)	21–22 weeks	52.01 ± 3.9	67.22 ± 9.02	181.01 ± 15.31	178.79 ± 13.9	497.72 ± 138.03	20.99 ± 1.02
	33–35 weeks	82.77 ± 7.71	103.07 ± 8.33	299.82 ± 28.53	301.02 ± 29.34	2607.7 ± 631.0	22.73 ± 1.38

Note: $p > 0.05$ for differences between groups.

Table 4. Ultrasound-fetometry data in pregnant women vaccinated against influenza (M ± m).

Parameter		**Group I "MonoGrippol Plus" (n = 43)**	**Group II "Grippol® Plus" (n = 50)**	**Group III "Agrippal S1" (n = 48)**	**Group IV "Placebo" (n = 41)**
Women	Physiological birth	39 (90.7%)	48 (96.0%)	43 (89.5%)	35 (85.4%)
	Miscarriage	0	1 (2.0%)	1 (2.1%)	1 (2.4%)
	Premature birth	4 (9.3%)	1 (2.0%)	4 (8.3%)	3 (7.3%)
Infants	Without pathology	38 (88.4%)	46 (92.0%)	42 (87.5%)	33 (85.4%)
	Birth of babies with abnormalities or developmental defects	1 (2.3%)	1 (2.0%)	2 (4.2%)	2 (4.9%)
	Perinatal CNS lesions	4 (9.3%)	3 (6.0%)	5 (10.4%)	3 (7.3%)
	Intrauterine infection-like syndrome	2 (4.6%)	1 (2.0%)	4 (6.3%)	2 (4.9%)

Note: $p > 0.05$ for differences between groups.

Table 5. Outcomes of pregnancy and birth in women vaccinated against influenza.

II and III (85.4 and 92.9%, respectively) ($p > 0.05$). Further onwards, the number of infants receiving only breast milk gradually diminished (92.1% at 3 months and 65.8% at 6 months in group I; 85.4% at 3 months and 72.9% at 6 months in group II; 83.3% at 3 months and 69.0% at 6 months in group III; and 88.6% at 3 months and 60.0% at 6 months in group IV) ($p > 0.05$). Therefore, vaccination of women with subunit adjuvanted influenza vaccines during pregnancy has no further impact on lactation and duration of breastfeeding.

3.4.3. *Body weight and length*

Parameters of physical development of infants of the first 6 months of life from different groups were generally comparable. Body weight and body length at different time points were within the percentile rank (25-50-75). The Ketle 1 index in group I newborns was 65.1 ± 0.67, in group II—63.8 ± 1.22, in group III—65.5 ± 1.72, and in group IV—67.1 ± 1.03 ($p > 0.05$).

In the majority of cases, the proportionality of physical development among infants in their first few months of life had the average values of harmonious development, namely 65–74% in group I, 70–76% in group II, 69–81% in group III, and 69–76% in placebo group ($p > 0.05$). The infants with the average values below harmonious development were found equally often (14–22% in group I, 12–16% in group II, 12–19% in group III, and 18–21% in group IV). The infants with the average values above harmonious development (6–22% in group I, 10–17% in group II, 7–12% in group III, and 6–15% in group IV) were considered as a variant of body constitutional norm ($p > 0.05$). Infants with a disproportional physical development have not been found.

Therefore, our results attest to the sufficiency of basic criteria for infant development and reflect the population maturity in terms of their physical development regardless of vaccination of their mothers during pregnancy with different influenza subunit vaccines.

3.4.4. Neuropsychological development

Parameters of neuropsychological development (NPD) of children born to vaccinated mothers did not differ significantly from those of the placebo group. Overall, no changes of NPD have been observed in 81.6% of group I infants in their first 6 months of life who had been born to mothers vaccinated during pregnancy with a monovalent influenza vaccine. In other clinical groups, this parameter was 83.3% (group II), 78.6% (group III), and 77.1% (group IV) ($p > 0.05$). Within the structure of occasional NPD disorders, there were conditions which number did not exceed the average statistical rate of neurological pathology in a given pediatric age group.

It was noted that infants born to women vaccinated during pregnancy with trivalent influenza vaccines were 1.8-times less likely to develop non-influenza respiratory infections within the first 6 months of life as compared to infants from placebo control group (**Figure 2**).

3.5. Immunogenicity of adjuvanted influenza vaccine "Grippol® Plus" in pregnant women vaccinated during different trimesters of pregnancy

In this study, the level of post-vaccination antibodies to influenza virus was evaluated only in a group of pregnant women and non-pregnant women vaccinated with a trivalent adjuvanted influenza vaccine with the aim of revealing the features of the effect of pregnancy on the synthesis of antibodies. Since it has been already proven that the introduction of subunit unadjuvanted vaccines in pregnant women is accompanied by the formation of antibodies to the influenza virus in values not differing from those in non-pregnant ones, it seemed to us interesting to investigate the interaction of the immunoadjuvant preparation with the transiently altered immune status of the pregnant woman [36].

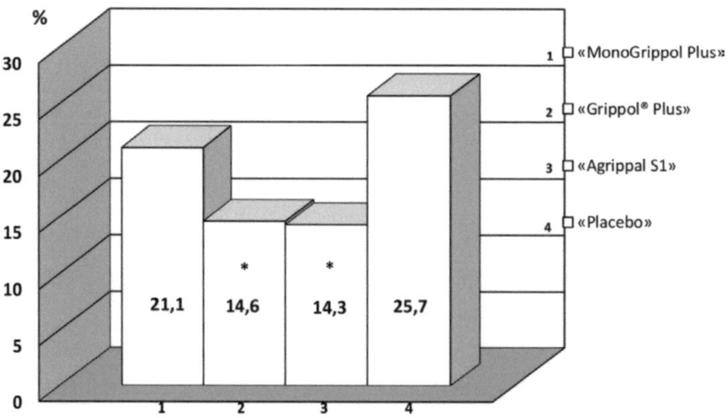

Figure 2. Incidence of morbidity due to non-influenza respiratory infections in infants during their first 6 months of life. *Note:* *- $p < 0.05$ for differences between groups I, II, III and group IV.

It was found that a part of women before immunization had a seroprotective (≥1:40) baseline antibody level to vaccine strains of influenza virus (**Table 6**). In all examined women, the antibody titer was higher to influenza virus B (22.2% of women in the second trimester, 26.1% in the third trimester and 25.7% in non-pregnant women). This is probably due to the duration of its circulation in the population and the formation of natural immunity. It should be noted that none of the participants in the study was vaccinated before and did not confirm an acute illness caused by the influenza virus. One month after vaccination, women of all groups demonstrated a significant rise in antibody titer that fully met one of the CPMP criteria. In the post-vaccination period, the antiviral antibody titer gradually declined reaching a significant difference against baseline by 3 months postpartum in women vaccinated in the second and third trimesters. The observed difference referred only to viral strain A/H1N1/v ($p < 0.05$). It is possible that the loss of antibodies to a pandemic strain is associated with the peculiarities of the formation of immunity after its first administration. Other authors have shown that specific antibodies to this strain in the post-vaccination period can be synthesized at lower values and therefore be accompanied by their faster loss. At 6 and 12 months post-vaccination, there was a marked regression of seroprotection level with regard to antibody titer against strains A/H1N1/v, A/H3N2/and B in women vaccinated during pregnancy in the second and third trimesters ($p < 0.01$). Such trend was also traced in a group of non-pregnant women; however, the changes were less remarkable, with a fairly significant fraction of subjects having a high level of protective antibodies. Similar dynamics of post-vaccination antibodies were noted in pregnant women vaccinated with subunit non-adjuvanted influenza vaccine [37].

The rate of development and intensity of protective immunity include the level and factor of seroconversion across all influenza virus strains. Those were compared between the groups, and it was found that their values met the CPMP criteria (**Table 7**). The majority of data obtained did not differ between the groups. One exception was the seroconversion factor for strain B in pregnant women vaccinated in the third trimester of pregnancy (5.1) when it was compared with the matching parameter in the non-pregnant women group (6.9) ($p < 0.05$).

The dynamics of influenza antibody (AB) titers based on the geometric mean titer (GMT) reflect the decline of antibody level with time in the post-vaccination period (**Table 8**). It was noted that at one month post-vaccination, the value of GMT AB to A/H1N1/v strain in women vaccinated in the second trimester of pregnancy was significantly lower (49.12 ± 0.29) compared to subjects vaccinated in the third trimester of pregnancy (60.99 ± 0.25) ($p < 0.05$). During all subsequent periods, this parameter showed no differences with regard to the trimester of pregnancy.

Pregnant women vaccinated in the third trimester of pregnancy showed at 3 months post-vaccination and throughout the follow-up period lower GMT AB titers to strain B compared to the non-pregnant women ($p < 0.05$ to $p < 0.01$). Similar trend was traced in women of the same group with regard to all influenza virus strains at 6 months postpartum compared to the non-pregnant women ($p < 0.05$ to $p < 0.01$).

Therefore, the post-vaccination immune response in women vaccinated with a trivalent adjuvanted influenza vaccine at different times of pregnancy, during the first month, did not differ

	Periods of observation	Second trimester (n = 27)			Third trimester (n = 23)			Non-pregnant women (n = 19)		
		A/H1N1/v	A/H3N2/	B	A/H1N1/v	A/H3N2/	B	A/H1N1/v	A/H3N2/	B
Seroprotection level (AB titer ≥ 1:40) (%)	Before vaccination (V)	3.7	11.1	22.2	8.7	13.0	26.1	2.6	14.1	25.7
	1 month post-V	77.0*	88.9*	85.2*	87.0*	87.0*	91.3*	83.1*	90.2*	94.4*
	3 months post-V	74.8	88.4	84.2	—	—	—	80.6	88.7	92.0
	6 (3) months post-V 2–3 days postpartum	74.1	81.5	77.8	62.0	76.2	71.4	78.5	83.1	88.2
	9 (6) months post-V 3 months postpartum	57.7 ×	69.2	65.4	57.1 ×	71.4	62.0	71.4	78.6	72.8
	12 (9) months post-V 6 months postpartum	48.2 ∇∇/×	65.4 ∇∇	57.7 ∇∇/×	50.0 ∇∇/×	61.1 ∇∇	55.6 ∇∇/×	67.6 ∇	72.5 ∇	69.1 ∇∇

Note: Time period elapsed since the moment of vaccination of women in the third trimester of pregnancy (group II) is given in brackets.

*: $p < 0.01$—the intra-group difference for the second/third trimesters of pregnancy; non-pregnant in-between pre-vaccination and 1 month post-vaccination.

∇: $p < 0.05$; ∇∇: $p < 0.01$—the intra-group difference for the second/third trimesters of pregnancy; non-pregnant in-between 1 month and 12 (9) months post-vaccination.

×: $p < 0.05$; ××: $p < 0.01$—difference between the second/third trimesters of pregnancy group and non-pregnant group.

Table 6. Seroprotection level in pregnant women vaccinated with "Grippol® Plus," allowing for trimester of pregnancy.

http://dx.doi.org/10.5772/intechopen.69271

Parameter	Second trimester (n = 27)			Third trimester (n = 23)			Non-pregnant women (n = 19)		
	A/H1N1/	A/H3N2/	B	A/H1N1/	A/H3N2/	B	A/H1N1/	A/H3N2/	B
Seroconversion level (%)	70.4	77.8	74.1	69.6	78.3	65.2	71.5	81.1	70.3
Seroconversion factor	6.5	7.2	6.5	7.1	6.5	5.1*	6.8	7.6	6.9

Note: *$p < 0.05$ for difference between the third trimester group and non-pregnant group.

Table 7. Seroconversion level and seroconversion factor in pregnant women vaccinated with "Grippol® Plus," allowing for the trimester.

	Periods of observation	Second trimester (n = 27)			Third trimester (n = 23)			Non-pregnant (n = 19)		
		A/H1N1/v	A/H3N2/	B	A/H1N1/v	A/H3N2/	B	A/H1N1/v	A/H3N2/	B
Geometric mean antibody titer (log_2GMT AB)	Before vaccination (V)	7.54 ± 0.17	8.79 ± 0.23	13.96 ± 0.26	8.60 ± 0.23	10.62 ± 0.24	14.36 ± 0.25	8.02 ± 0.15	9.12 ± 0.21	14.19 ± 0.21
	1 month post-V	49.12 ± 0.29	63.49 ± 0.28	90.96 ± 0.36	60.99 ± 0.25 *	68.81 ± 0.26	73.08 ± 0.24	52.12 ± 0.22	59.47 ± 0.24	81.11 ± 0.37
	3 months post-V	47.87 ± 0.27	55.85 ± 0.26	65.15 ± 0.35	—	—	—	51.31 ± 0.24	57.73 ± 0.31	73.88 ± 0.26
	6 (3) months post-V 2–3 days postpartum	41.04 ± 0.23	44.33 ± 0.22	47.87 ± 0.32	41.34 ± 0.30	45.64 ± 0.25	42.72 ± 0.30 ×	48.56 ± 0.22	55.53 ± 0.24	63.13 ± 0.36
	9 (6) months post-V 3 months postpartum	30.64 ± 0.23	29.83 ± 0.22 ××	32.32 ± 0.29	30.72 ± 0.31	31.75 ± 0.32 ×	26.92 ± 0.35 ××	44.82 ± 0.25	51.79 ± 0.23	57.71 ± 0.31
	12 (9) months post-V 6 months postpartum	21.67 ± 0.24 ∇∇/×	24.10 ± 0.26 ∇∇/××	25.42 ± 0.25 ∇∇/××	20.79 ± 0.34 ∇∇/×	25.19 ± 0.33 ∇∇/××	19.24 ± 0.35 ∇∇/××	38.17 ± 0.26 ∇	44.47 ± 0.21 ∇	50.03 ± 0.28 ∇∇

Note: Time period elapsed since the moment of vaccination of women in the third trimester of pregnancy is given in brackets.

*: $p < 0.05$—for difference between the second trimester/third trimester groups.

∇: $p < 0.05$; ∇∇: $p < 0.01$—the intra-group difference for the second/third trimesters of pregnancy; non-pregnant between 1 month and 12 (9) months post-vaccination.

×: $p < 0.05$; ××: $p < 0.01$—for difference between the second trimester group, third trimester group and non-pregnant group.

Table 8. Geometric mean antibody titer in pregnant women vaccinated with "Grippol® Plus," allowing for the trimester.

from that in vaccinated non-pregnant women and fully met the CPMP criteria. The level of antibodies to strain A/H1N1/v following administration of a trivalent vaccine was nearly the same as with vaccination of pregnant women with the monovalent, subunit, adjuvanted vaccine [38, 39]

With time the postpartum women demonstrated a more pronounced reduction of seroprotection level, especially against the A/H1N1/v strain. After 6 months postpartum, the rate of regression of seroprotection level in subgroups of vaccinated pregnant women (taking into account the gestational age) has increased 1.6–1.7-fold (A/H1N1/v), 1.4-fold (A/H3N2) and 1.5- to 1.6-fold (B), whereas in the non-pregnant women group same parameter was 1.2-fold (A/H1N1/v), 1.2-fold (A/H3N2) and 1.4-fold (B), respectively. This trend was in line with dynamic reduction of the MGT AB values during the last months of the follow-up [38]. Consequently, the existing physiological immunological changes in the immune system during pregnancy may affect the formation and preservation of post-vaccination antibodies to strains of influenza virus when using subunit immunoadjuvant vaccines. However, this assumption should be confirmed by new data research.

3.6. Immunologic effectiveness of vaccination of pregnant women using "Grippol® Plus" influenza vaccine in mother-infant pairs

Analysis of transplacental immunity in the first months of life of infants born to women vaccinated during pregnancy with "Grippol® Plus" vaccine has shown that the level of seroprotection against influenza virus strains significantly differed only in the mother-infant pairs from the group of subjects vaccinated in the second trimester of pregnancy ($p < 0.05$), while no differences in the number of seroprotected infants have been found ($p > 0.05$) (**Table 9**). At 3 months after birth all infants, regardless of the time of their mothers' vaccination, demonstrated a significant reduction of protective titers of transplacental antibodies to vaccine strains of influenza virus as compared to their antibody titers obtained at birth and antibody titers in their mothers ($p < 0.01$). Further onwards, protective antibodies to vaccine strains of influenza virus completely vanished, and among the 6-month infants, the titer dropped to zero in both groups [40]. It should be noted that by 3 months of life, the rate of regression of antibody titer was higher in the subgroup of infants born to mothers vaccinated in late pregnancy, namely 2.8-fold higher for A/H1N1/v, 2.6-fold higher for A/H3N2/, and 4.0-fold higher for B strain.

Therefore, 52.3–61.9% of babies born to women vaccinated during pregnancy with "Grippol® Plus" vaccine had protective antibody levels against vaccine influenza strains at the time of their birth. This level of protection significantly declined with time and by 3 months of life remained at a protective level in only 14.2–24.0% of infants. At the age of 6 months, protective titers of maternal antibodies completely vanished in all infants. Infants born to women vaccinated in the second trimester of pregnancy had higher activity of protective antibodies and lower rate of reduction of seroprotection level which attests to a better preservation of the post-vaccination transplacental immunity. Thus, the advantage of vaccination of pregnant women with the use of immunoadjuvant subunit vaccine in the II trimester of gestation was revealed.

	Observation periods	Second trimester						Third trimester					
		A/H1N1/v		A/H3N2/		B		A/H1N1/v		A/H3N2/		B	
		M	**I**	**M**	**I**	**M**	**I**	**M**	**I**	**M**	**I**	**M**	**I**
Seroprotection level (%) (AB titer > 1:40)	Day 2–3 postpartum/ newborns	74.1	55.5 ×	81.5	59.3 ×	77.8	60.2 ×	62.0	52.3	76.2	61.9	71.4	57.1 ×
	At 3 months postpartum/3 months old	57.7	20.0 ××/⊗⊗	69.2	24.0 ××/⊗⊗	65.4	20.0 ▲××/⊗⊗	57.1	19.0 ××/⊗⊗	71.4	23.8 ××/⊗⊗	62.0	14.2 ××/⊗⊗
	At 6 months postpartum/6 months old	46.2	0 ⊗⊗	65.4	0 ⊗⊗	57.7	0 ⊗⊗	50.0	0 ⊗⊗	61.1	0 ⊗⊗	55.6	0 ⊗⊗
Geometric mean antibody titer (log_2GMT AB)	Day 2–3 postpartum/ newborns	41.04 ± 0.23	25.85 ± 0.29 ×	44.33 ± 0.22	27.22 ±0.26 ×	47.87 ±0.32	30.94 ±0.31	41.34 ±0.30	23.59 ±0.28 ×	45.64 ±0.25	26.91 ±0.25 ×	42.72 ±0.30	25.19 ±0.28 ×
	At 3 months postpartum/3 months old	30.64 ± 0.23	11.30 ± 0.26 ××/⊗⊗	29.83 ± 0.22	13.86 ±0.24 ××/⊗⊗	32.32 ±0.29	13.19 ±0.32 ××/⊗⊗	30.72 ±0.31	13.46 ±0.25 ××/⊗⊗	31.75 ±0.32	15.87 ±0.24 ××/⊗⊗	26.92 ±0.35	12.59 ±0.24 ××/⊗⊗
	At 6 months postpartum/6 months old	21.67 ± 0.24	7.52 ± 0.26 ××/⊗⊗	24.10 ± 0.26	8.49 ±0.20 ××/⊗⊗	25.42 ±0.25	7.23 ±0.22 ××/⊗⊗	20.79 ±0.34	8.91 ±0.20 ××/⊗⊗	25.19 ±0.33	11.22 ±0.19 ××/⊗⊗	19.24 ±0.35	7.94 ±0.18 ××/⊗⊗

Note: **M**—mother; **I**—infant.

▲: $p < 0.05$—for differences between infants from different observation groups.

×: $p < 0.05$; ××: $p < 0.01$—for differences between "mother-infant" groups.

⊗: $p < 0.05$; ⊗⊗: $p < 0.01$—for infants' intra-group differences versus at birth data.

Table 9. State of transplacental post-vaccination immunity in "mother-infant" pairs following vaccination against influenza using "Grippol® Plus" vaccine.

4. Conclusions

1. Different underlying diseases diagnosed in women of reproductive age are not an impediment to influenza vaccination during pregnancy.
2. Influenza vaccination during pregnancy using Russian-made polymer-subunit monovalent and trivalent vaccines ("MonoGrippol Plus" and "Grippol® Plus") in 58.1–60.0% of cases is accompanied by asymptomatic post-vaccination period. The frequency of systemic (generalized) post-vaccination reactions in immunized women (6.9–14.0%) does not differ significantly from that in placebo control group (10.2–12.2%).
3. Administration of adjuvanted vaccines to pregnant women does not cause disturbances of their metabolic homeostasis, hormonal profile, and cytokine profile.
4. Vaccination of pregnant women against influenza does not affect trophoblast function and fetal growth. Vaccination neither bears the risk of miscarriage nor influences the pattern and duration of breastfeeding.
5. Considering that safety of adjuvanted influenza vaccines has been proven by clinical and laboratory investigations, additional safety studies in pregnant women before and post-vaccination are redundant.
6. Babies born to mothers vaccinated against influenza with adjuvanted vaccines ("MonoGrippol Plus" and "Grippol® Plus") have a high level of physiological maturity. The basic parameters of physical and neuropsychological development in the early postnatal period in such infants do not differ from those of infants from control group.
7. Infants born to women vaccinated during pregnancy with influenza vaccines are 1.8 times less likely to develop non-influenza respiratory infections within the first 6 months of life as compared to infants born to unvaccinated mothers.
8. Administration of adjuvanted trivalent vaccine to pregnant women elicits a pronounced immune response to influenza vaccine strains A and B that fully meets the CPMP criteria for seroprotection levels: A/H1N1/v—82.0%, A/H3N2/—88.0% and B—88.3%.
9. Women vaccinated with the polymer-subunit vaccine in the second trimester of pregnancy benefit from higher seroprotection level and longer retention time of influenza-specific antibodies.
10. Protective titers of transplacental antibodies to different influenza virus strains are found in 52.3–68.9% of infants that is comparable to control figures. Higher levels of protective antibodies to different influenza virus strains are found in infants whose mothers have been vaccinated with adjuvanted vaccine "Grippol® Plus" in the second trimester of pregnancy.
11. Analysis of mother-infant pairs showed a direct correlation in levels of post-vaccination IgG influenza-specific antibodies between mother and infant. However, after 3 months, protective antibodies to influenza virus strains were detectable in 14.2–36.1% of infants followed by their complete disappearance at 6 months of life versus 57.1–71.4% (3 months)

and 48.1–65.4% (6 months) in their mothers. This observation provides substantiation that vaccination against influenza in high-risk infants shall start at the age of 6 months.

12. The results obtained allow us to recommend the "Grippol® Plus" vaccine for use in healthcare practice for specific prevention of seasonal influenza in pregnant women and their offspring up to age 6 months inclusive, using a single-dose vaccination schedule.

Author details

Kostinov Mikhail Petrovich[1,2], Cherdantsev Alexander Petrovich[3], Shmitko Anna Dmitrievna[1], Akhmatova Nelly Kimovna[1], Kostinova Aristitsa Mikhailovna[4], Praulova Darya Alexandrovna[5], Polyschuk Valentina Borisovna[1], Protasov Andrey Dmitrievich[6*], Zhestkov Alexander Victorovich[6] and Tezikov Yuriy Vladimirovich[7]

*Address all correspondence to: crosss82@mail.ru

1 Federal State-Funded Research Institution "Scientific Research Institute of Vaccines and Sera named after I.I. Mechnikov", Moscow, Russia

2 Federal State-Funded Educational Institution of Higher Education "First Moscow State Medical University named after I.M. Sechenov" of Ministry of Healthcare of Russia, Moscow, Russia

3 Federal State-Funded Educational Institution of Higher Education "Ulyanovsk State University", Ulyanovsk, Russia

4 National Research Center–Institute of Immunology Federal Medical-Biological Agency of Russia, Moscow, Russia

5 Dmitriy Rogachev Federal Research Center of Pediatric Hematology, Oncology and Immunology of the Ministry of Health of Russian Federation, Moscow, Russia

6 Federal State-Funded Educational Institution of Higher Education "Samara State Medical University" of Ministry of Healthcare of Russia, Samara, Russia

7 Department of Obstetrics and Gynecology №1, Samara State Medical University, Samara, Russia

References

[1] ECDC scientific advice on seasonal influenza vaccination of children and pregnant women: ECDC Technical report/European Centre for Disease Prevention and Control. Stockholm: ECDC. 2012. 68

[2] Jamieson DJ, et al. H1N1 2009 influenza virus infection during pregnancy in the USA. Lancet. 2009;**374**. P. 451-458

[3] Tarbaeva DA, Kostinov MP, Zagorodnya E D, Josefson SA, Cherdantsev AP. Obstetrical and perinatal outcomes of pregnancy complicated with acute respiratory infection in the second trimester of pregnancy. Obstetrics and Gynecology (Russian). 2012. (2). pp. 67-71

[4] Tarbaeva DA, Kostinov MP, Josefson SA, Zagorodnya E D. Clinical course and outcomes of influenza A (HINI) 2009 infection in pregnant women. Journal of Microbiology, Epidemiology and Immunobiology (Russian). 2011;(4):pp. 71-76

[5] Mullooly JP. Risk of acute respiratory disease among pregnant women during influenza A epidemics [Text]. Mullooly JP, Barker WH, Nolan TF. Public Health Reports. 1986. Vol. 101:pp. 205-211

[6] Fiore AE. Prevention and control of influenza with vaccines: Recommendations of the advisory committee on immunization practices (ACIP). 2010. Fiore AE. et al. MMWR Recommendations and Reports. 2010;Vol. 59: pp. 1-62

[7] Zaman K, et al. Effectiveness of maternal influenza immunisation in mothers and infants. The New England Journal of Medicine. 2008;**359**(15):pp. 1555-1564

[8] Englund JA. Maternal immunization with inactivated influenza vaccine: Rationale and experience. Vaccine. 2003;**21**:pp. 3460-3464

[9] Fiore AE, et al. Prevention and control of influenza with vaccines: Recommendations of the advisory committee on immunization practices (ACIP). MMWR Recommendations and Reports. 2010;(59):pp. 1-62

[10] CDC. Guidelines for Vaccinating Pregnant Women: From Recommendations of the Advisory Committee on Immunization Practices (ACIP) [Electronic resource]. Centers for Disease Control and Prevention. 2007. Mode of access: http://www.cdc.gOv/vaccines/pubs/preg-guide.htm#5/

[11] Zverev VV, Kostinov MP, Cherdantsev AP, Kuselman AI, Kiselev OI, Erofeeva MK, Krasnopolskiy VI, Novikova S V, Serova OF, Briko NI, Chuchalin AG. Vaccination of Pregnant Women Against Influenza: Federal Clinical Guidelines. Moscow (Russian). 2015. p. 42

[12] Cherdantsev AP, Kostinov MP, Kuselman AI. Vaccine Prophylaxis of Influenza in Pregnant Women. Manual for Physicians. M. 4Mpress (Russian). 2013. p. 96

[13] Cherdantsev AP, Kostinov MP, Kuselman AI. Vaccine prophylaxis of influenza in pregnant women/Manual for physicians. 2nd edition with supplement. M. MDV Art Studio «Constellation» (Russian). 2014. p. 112

[14] Tsai T, et al. Exposure to MF59-adjuvanted influenza vaccines during pregnancy–retrospective analysis. Vaccine. 2010;**7**(28):pp. 1877-1880

[15] Kostinov MP, Kostinova TA, Zolotareva TA. Potentials of vaccination against influenza in high-risk patient groups. «Hospital physician» Journal (Russian). 2001;(10). pp.52-54

[16] Clinico-immunologic effectiveness of immunobiological preparations/Reference book. Kostinov MP, Ozeretskovsky NA. Eds. Moscow. 2004–«Miklosh» (Russian). p. 256

[17] Kostinov MP, Lavrov VF. New generation vaccines for the prevention of infectious diseases. 2nd edition, with supplement, M.: MDV (Russian). 2010. p. 192

[18] Chebykina AV, Kostinov MP, Magarshak OO. Evaluation of safety and effectiveness of vaccination against influenza in patients with syndrome of bronchial obstruction. Epidemiology and Vaccinoprophylaxis (Russian). 2010;**6**(55): pp. 50-53

[19] Protasov AD, Zhestkov AV, Lavrentyeva NE, Kostinov MP, Ryzhov AA. Effect of complex vaccination against pneumococcal, haemophilus type B and influenza infections in patients with chronic obstructive pulmonary disease. Journal of Microbiology. Epidemiology and Immunobiology (Russian). 2011;(4):pp. 80-84

[20] Kostinov MP, Yerofeeva MK, Kharit SM. Effectiveness and safety of influenza vaccinoprophylaxis in different populations. All-Russia Interdisciplinary Journal TERRA MEDICA® (Russian). 2011;(2):pp. 7-11

[21] Kostinov MP, Chuchalin AG, Chebykina AV. Particulars of formation of post-vaccination immunity to influenza in patients with chronic broncho-pulmonary pathology. Infectious Diseases (Russian). 2011;**9**(3):pp. 35-40

[22] Vaccination of adults with broncho-pulmonary pathology. Manual for physicians (Kostinov MP., Ed.), M: 2013. Art studio «Constellation» (Russian). p. 109

[23] Vaccination of Children with Impaired Health State. Manual for Physicians (Kostinov MP, Ed.), 4th edition, M.: 4Mpress (Russian). 2013. p. 432

[24] Vaccines and Vaccination. National Manual (brief version, Zverev VV, Khaitov RM, Eds.) M.: Publishing group «GEOTAR-Media» (Russian). 2014: p. 640

[25] Cherdantsev AP. Effectiveness of immunoadjuvanted vaccines against influenza in pregnant women and evaluation of their safety for fetus and newborn/D. Med. Sci. Thesis (Russian), Moscow. 2013: p. 39

[26] Cherdantsev AP, Kuselman AI, Sinitsyna MN, Shalyagina ME, Kostinov MP, Tarbaeva DA. Study of clinical safety of vaccination against influenza in pregnant women. Medical Almanac (Russian). 2011;**4**(17):pp. 120-122

[27] Kostinov MP, Cherdantsev AP, Savisco AA, Tarbaeva DA, Solovieva IL. True and false reactions to influenza vaccine in pregnant women. Problems of Gynecology, Obstetrics and Perinatology (Russian). 2011;**10**(6):pp. 44-48

[28] Serova OF, Semenova SS, Cherdantsev AP, Tsaregorodseva MV. Evaluation of clinic-laboratory parameters in pregnant women vaccinated against influenza. Russian herald of obstetrics and gynecology (Russian). 2015;(2):pp. 75-79

[29] Cherdantsev AP, Kostinov MP, Kuselman AI, Voznesenskaya NV. Vaccination of pregnant women against influenza A(HINI). Journal of microbiology, epidemiology and immunobiology (Russian). 2011;(4):pp. 46-50

[30] Kostinov MP, Cherdantsev AP, Semenova SS, Tarbaeva DA, Savisco AA, Serova OF, Josefson S A, Akhmatova NK, Kostinova TA, Praulova DA. Obstetrical and perinatal

outcomes after vaccination against influenza or past respiratory infection. Gynecology (Russian), 2015;**14**(3):pp. 43-46

[31] Kostinov MP, Cherdantsev AP. Clinical and immunological safety of inactivated, immunoadjuvanted, subunit vaccine against influenza in pregnant women. Obstetrics and Gynecology (Russian). 2016;(2):pp. 64-69

[32] Cherdantsev AP, Kostinov MP, Kuselman AI, Liutaya ZA, Kutbutdinova MH. Analysis of the ante- and postnatal development of infants against a background of vaccination of pregnant women against influenza. Russian Herald of Perinatology and Pediatrics (Russian). 2013;**58**(2):pp. 30-34

[33] Cherdantsev AP, Kuselman AI, Kostinov MP, Liutaya ZA, Deryabina EV, Azizova R Sh, Melnik RH. Postnatal development of infants born to mothers vaccinated against influenza. Ulyanovsk Medico-Biological Journal (Russian). 2012;(3):pp.80-84

[34] Kostinov MP, Cherdantsev AP, Praulova DA, Kostinova AM. Vaccination against influenza—A safe way to protect pregnant women and newborns from consequences of infection. Russian herald of perinatology and pediatrics (Russian). 2015;(5):pp. 69-74

[35] Kostinov MP, Cherdantsev AP. State of health of infants born to mothers vaccinated against influenza during pregnancy. Pediatrics. Journal named after G.N. Speransky (Russian). 2016;(195):pp. 67-71

[36] Kostinov MP, Khromova EA, Savisko AA, Kostinova AM. Features of the immune system functioning during physiological pregnancy and their relationship with vaccination against influenza. CONSILIUM MEDICUM (Russian). 2016;#6.;**18**. pp. 59-62

[37] Mikhail P. Kostinov, Alexander P. Cherdantsev, Anna D Shmitko, Dmitry Pakhomov, Evgenia O Demina. Duration of Preservation of Antibodies to the Flu Virus in the Mother-Child Pairs during the Vaccination of Women Depending on the Trimester of Pregnancy. International Journal of Biomedicine. 2015;**5**(4): 179-183

[38] Kostinov MP, Cherdantsev AP, Briko NI. Mono and trivalent immunoadjuvant influenza vaccines immunologenicity and safety in pregnant women, The Fifth International Conference & Exhibitiom on: Influenza Vaccines for the World, 6-9 October, Albufeira Algarve Portugal, 2015. Posters № 109

[39] Cherdantsev AP, Kostinov MP, Kuselman AI, Dagil Yu A, Savisko AA. Post-vaccination immunity to influenza virus A/California/2009(H1N1)v in immunized pregnant women. Medical Immunology (Russian). 2012;**14**(6): pp. 527-532

[40] Kostinov MP, Cherdantsev AP and Pakhomov DV. Anti-influenza antibody level in mother-infant pairs depending on trimester of vaccination of pregnant women using immunoadjivant vaccine. Vaccines. 2015;**6**:5. http://dx.doi.org/2157-7560.1000297

Section 4

Biotechnological Approaches to Vaccine Production

Chapter 5

Biotechnologies Applied in Biomedical Vaccines

Yuan-Chuan Chen, Hwei-Fang Cheng,
Yi-Chen Yang and Ming-Kung Yeh

Additional information is available at the end of the chapter

http://dx.doi.org/10.5772/intechopen.69547

Abstract

Vaccination, the administration of an antigenic material (vaccine), is considered to be the most effective method for disease prevention and control. A vaccine usually contains an agent that resembles a diseases-causing pathogen and is often made from inactivated microbes, live attenuated microbes, its toxins, or part of surface antigens (subunit). However, the modern biotechnological tools and genomics have opened a new era to develop novel vaccines and many products are successfully marketing around the world. It is important to formulate and deliver these vaccines appropriately to maximize the potential advances in prevention, therapy, and vaccinology. New vaccines employing biotechnological innovations are helping us to change the way for illness prevention. The clinical application of vaccines will be diversified along with the development of biotechnologies. In modern society, the outbreak of many infectious diseases has decreased through vaccination, but the burden of noninfectious diseases is growing. The new biotechnologies may result in not only the appreciation of vaccines which are critical in inducing protection against an infectious disease but also the production of therapeutic vaccines which are effective for alldiseases including infectious and noninfectious diseases.

Keywords: biotechnology, vaccine, genetic engineering, prevention, therapy

1. Introduction

A vaccine is a biological preparation that provides active acquired immunity to a particular pathogen. The agent stimulates the immune system to recognize itself as a foreign threat and thus destroys and remembers it, so that the immune system can easily destroy any of these pathogens when they later invade into the body. The following vaccine characteristics may be altered or enhanced by biotechnologies.

1.1. Type

Inactivated microbes, live attenuated microbes, toxoids, and subunits have been manufactured as vaccines and employed to trigger adaptive immune responses [1].

1.2. Mode of action

The process is an artificial induction of immunity with an effort to protect against infectious diseases by priming the immune system with an immunogen. Vaccination traditionally includes various ways of administration such as given by injection, oral, intranasal, and percutaneous administration.

1.3. Effectiveness

The efficacy of vaccines is dependent on a number of factors such as the disease itself, the strain of vaccine, the vaccination schedule, idiosyncratic response to vaccination, and assorted factors, such as ethnicity, age, or genetic predisposition.

1.4. Potency

The potency is critically correlated to vaccine quality and efficacy. Its assay methods are variable, including *in vivo* assay, such as mice challenge test, plaque reduction neutralization test (PRNT), and *in vitro* assay, such as enzyme-linked immunosorbent assay (ELISA).

1.5. Safety

Vaccines are one of the safest medical products, but they are sometimes risky. The safety should be evaluated in clinical phases and postmarket surveillance. Accurate information about the value of vaccines as well as their possible side effects helps people to make decisions about vaccination.

2. Biotechnology

Biotechnology is the technological application of biological organisms, systems, and processes to develop, make, or modify products for specific uses such as pharmaceuticals, crops, and livestock. It encompasses a wide range of procedures for modifying living organisms according to human purposes. Traditional methods are the employment of artificial selection and hybridization, but modern usage also includes genetic engineering as well as cell and tissue culture technologies. In this section, we review some biotechnologies applied for the development and production of vaccines.

2.1. Application

Biotechnology is mainly used in three ways as follows: separation of a pure antigen using a specific monoclonal antibody; synthesis of an antigen with the assistance of a cloned gene; and synthesis of peptides to be used as vaccines.

2.2. Approach

2.2.1. Reverse vaccinology

The basic idea of reverse vaccinology is that an entire pathogenic genome can be sequenced and screened by employing bioinformatics methods to explore genes. Functional genomics approaches, such as DNA microarrays, proteomics, and comparative genome analysis, are used for the identification of virulence factors and novel vaccine candidates. This new computational approach allows prediction of all antigens, independent of their abundance and immunogenicity during infection. The first attempt at reverse vaccinology began with *Meningococcus* B (MenB) vaccine. Moreover, it has been used on several other bacterial vaccines such as antibiotic-resistant *Staphylococcus aureus* and *Streptococcus pneumoniae* [2].

Reverse vaccinology have changed the concepts and approaches for vaccine candidate selection and design. Genome investigation and selection of antigens provide a new way to study the pathogenesis mechanisms. The resulting lists of novel candidates which reveal new aspects of pathogenesis will promote the rational design of optimal vaccine antigens. Applying genomic approaches to study both hosts and pathogens will ultimately drive and guide next-generation vaccine design [3].

2.2.2. Recombinant subunit vaccination

The gene cloning is a powerful tool to synthesize protein materials to subunit vaccine by recombinant DNA techniques. Recombinant subunit vaccines are made from a fragment of protein (antigen) expressed in the laboratory using the viral DNA, for example, hepatitis B (HB) vaccine. The hepatitis B virus (HBV) gene that codes for the antigen is inserted into baker's yeast genome and then expresses the antigen protein. The antigen protein is harvested and purified to be used for the vaccine. This technique is also being used to explore a vaccine against hepatitis C [4].

Recombinant-DNA techniques can facilitate the development of new principles to design and produce subunit vaccines. The recombinant subunit vaccine can furthermore be adapted by gene-fusion technology, to be efficiently incorporated into immunopotentiating adjuvant systems. The recombinant strategies have become increasingly important to the passive vaccination strategy and use antibodies or antibody fragments to prevent infectious diseases [5].

2.2.3. Recombinant protein vaccination

Upon infection, a pathogen produces proteins to elicit an immune response from the infected body. The gene encoding such a protein is isolated from the causative organism and used to develop a recombinant DNA which is expressed in a heterologous expression system (e.g., bacterium, yeast, or insect). Recombinant protein vaccines, such as cholera vaccine, diphtheria toxoid, and tetanus toxoid, are composed of protein/toxin antigens that have either been produced in another host organism or purified from large amount of pathogens. The vaccinated persons produce antibodies to the protein/toxin antigen to protect themselves from diseases.

The baculovirus-insect cell expression system is also a recombinant protein manufacturing platform for the production of complex proteins. The technology is used for the mass production of various recombinant protein vaccines. The major advantage is that a universal "plug and play" process may be used to produce a variety of protein-based prophylactic and therapeutic vaccines for human uses [6].

2.2.4. Deoxyribonucleic acid (DNA) vaccination

DNA vaccination is a technique for protecting against diseases through the direct injection of genetically engineered DNA. The gene responsible for the immunogenic protein is cloned with a corresponding expression vector. This DNA will trigger an immune response and the individual is successfully vaccinated. DNA vaccines may have the ability to induce a wider range of immune response types over conventional vaccines.

Despite several DNA vaccines are available for veterinary uses, none of them is commercial for human uses. Research is being investigated using the approach for controlling infectious diseases and several cancers in humans. For instance, a synthetic consensus antispike protein DNA vaccine induces protective immunity against Middle East respiratory syndrome (MERS) coronavirus in nonhuman primates [7]. The improved formulations and delivery methods can increase the uptake of vaccine plasmids by cells. The optimization of vaccine vectors and encoded antigens, and the adding of novel adjuvants potentially increase and direct the host immune responses. Therefore, current DNA vaccines may induce more potent, cellular, and humoral immune responses to be tested for both preventative and therapeutic uses [8].

2.2.5. Messenger ribonucleic acid (mRNA) vaccination

mRNA vaccines consist of mRNA, which is encoded by antigen genes of an infectious agent. When the mRNA is administered into host cells, it will translate protein antigens that elicit protective immunity against the infectious agent [9]. Vaccines based on mRNA may offer a solution as sequence-matched, clinical-grade material could allow quick responses to the emergence of pandemic microbe strains.

mRNA vaccines have an outstanding safety profile and the unmet genetic flexibility. mRNA vaccines can induce a balanced immune response comprising both cellular and humoral immunity. Compared with DNA vaccines, mRNA offers stronger safety advantages in which it harbors only the elements directly required for expression of the encoded protein and hardly interacts with the genome [10]. Because any protein can be encoded and expressed by mRNA without the need to adjust the production process, mRNA vaccines offer maximum flexibility with respect to vaccine production, and principally enable the development of prophylactic and therapeutic vaccines fighting against infections and cancers [10].

2.3. Advantages

(1) Low risk for infection: Recombinant vaccines do not contain actual pathogens; only parts of the microbes (DNA, RNA, or protein) are used for making vaccines. Thus, recombinant

vaccines are safer than conventional vaccines and can be given to people with weakened immune systems.

(2) Induction of more efficient immunity: Recombinant vaccines potentially induce both humoral and cellular immune responses to result in more effective vaccination.

2.4. Challenges

(1) Complex vaccination schedules: The vaccines produced by biotechnologies are usually only parts of microbes (DNA, RNA, or protein); therefore, it is required to have multiple doses for maximum effectiveness either to produce sufficient initial immune responses or to boost responses that fade over time. To achieve full immunity, several doses must be given to induce additional "booster" shots for proper long-term immunity.

(2) Economics: The research and development (R&D) of vaccines using biotechnologies is risky, costly, and time consuming. Most pharmaceutical firms and vaccine manufacturers have little incentive to develop vaccines based on biotechnologies because of limited revenue.

3. Products

Many products based on biotechnologies have been successfully marketing in many countries for years (**Table 1**).

3.1. Hepatitis B virus (HBV) vaccine: Recombivax HB®, Engerix-B®, Elovac B®, Genevac B®, and Shanvac B®

The vaccine is designed to prevent hepatitis B and currently produced with recombinant DNA techniques. It contains one of the viral envelope proteins-hepatitis B surface antigens (HBsAg) and produced in yeast cells, into which the genetic code for HBsAg has been inserted. The

Product	**Recombivax HB®, Engerix B®, Elovac B®, Genevac B® Shanvac B®**	**Rotarix® RotaTeq®**	**Gardasil® Cervarix®**	**Dengvaxia®**	**Bexsero® Trumenba®**
Preventive infection	HBV	Rotavirus	HPV	Dengue virus	*Neisseria meningitidis* group B strain
Indication	Hepatitis B	Gastroenteritis	Cervical cancer	Dengue	Meningitis
Vaccine type	Subunit vaccine	Live attenuated vaccine	Subunit vaccine	Live attenuated vaccine	Subunit vaccine
Administration	IM	Oral	IM	IM	IM

Human papilloma virus (HPV); hepatitis B virus (HBV); and intramuscular injection (IM).

Table 1. Vaccine products based on biotechnologies (recombinant DNA technology).

antigen is harvested and purified from fermentation cultures of a recombinant strain of the yeast *Saccharomyces cerevisiae* containing the gene for the adw subtype of HBsAg [11, 12].

3.2. Rotavirus vaccine: Rotarix® and RotaTeq®

This vaccine is designed to protect against rotavirus infections that cause vomiting and severe diarrhea in infants and children. It contains live attenuated viruses and should not be given to people who are clinically immunosuppressed. Rotarix® is a monovalent and indicated for the prevention of rotavirus gastroenteritis caused by G1 and non-G1 types (G3, G4, and G9). RotaTeq® is a pentavalent vaccine that contains five rotavirus strains produced by reassortment. Four reassortant rotaviruses express one of the outer capsid, VP7, proteins (serotypes G1, G2, G3, or G4) from the human rotavirus parent strain and the attachment protein VP4 (type P7) from the bovine rotavirus parent strain [13, 14].

3.3. Human papilloma virus (HPV) vaccine: Gardasil® and Cervarix®

The vaccine is designed to prevent infection by certain types of HPV. HPV vaccines are subunit vaccines containing virus-like particles (VLPs) assembled from the major capsid protein (L1 protein) of HPV type 6, 11, 16, and 18 (GardasilTM) and type 16 and 18 (CervarixTM). Available vaccines protect against two or four types of HPV; however, all vaccines protect against at least HPV 16 and 18 that cause the greatest risk of cervical cancer. The L1 proteins of these HPV types (16 and 18) are separately produced using a recombinant baculovirus expression system and the insect cell line [15, 16].

3.4. Dengue vaccine: Dengvaxia® (CYD-TDV)

The vaccine is designed to induce an immune system to produce antibodies against four serotypes of dengue (DENV-1, 2, 3, and 4) and a live attenuated tetravalent chimeric vaccine using recombinant DNA technology by replacing the pre-membrane (PrM) and envelope (E) structural genes of the yellow fever live attenuated vaccine. For the vaccine, the virus is genetically engineered to include genes encoding for dengue proteins. Its production is based on a weakened combination of the yellow fever virus and each of the four virus serotypes [17–19].

3.5. Men B (*Neisseria meningitidis* group B strain) vaccine: Bexsero® and Trumenba®

The vaccine is indicated for active immunization to prevent invasive disease caused by *Neisseria meningitidis* serogroup B. The vaccine is manufactured using recombinant DNA technology (rDNA, component, adsorbed) and includes four antigenic proteins: Neisseria heparin binding antigen (NHBA), Neisserial adhesion A (NadA), Factor H binding protein (fHbp) and PorA to protect against the majority of circulating MenB strains [20].

4. Perspectives

In this section, we describe some trends for the development of vaccines using biotechnologies (**Figure 1**).

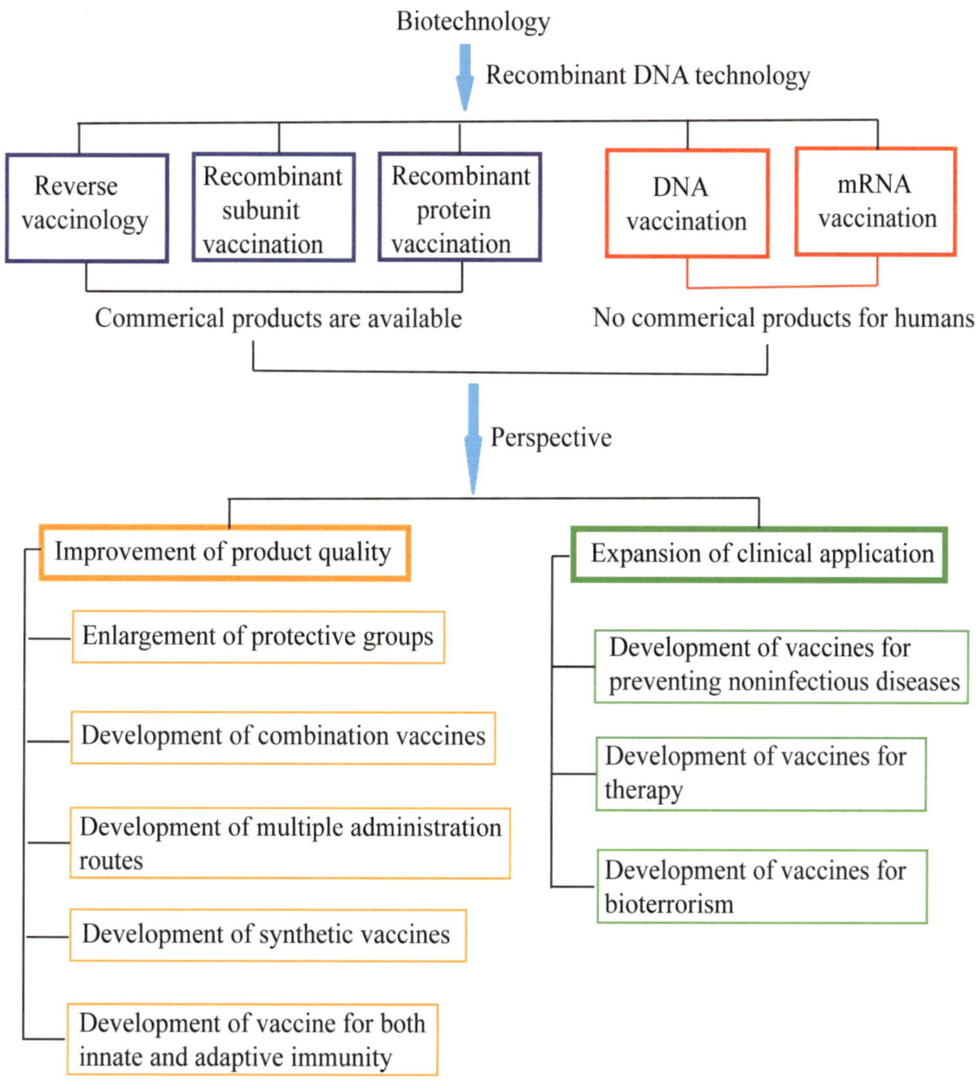

Figure 1. The perspectives of vaccine products based on biotechnologies.

4.1. Enlargement of protective groups

Most vaccines were focusing on infants and children, but adolescents and adults are gradually being targeted. During the course of their lives, adolescents and adults may need vaccination when they are hurt, sick, and pregnant or take a tour to some disease-endemic area. In addition, hospital patients, pregnant women, volunteer workers, individual with noninfectious diseases, and individual with chronic infections may need to prevent diseases necessarily than healthy persons; therefore, they will be the new target group for vaccination.

4.2. Development of combination vaccines

Combination vaccines include two or more vaccines that could be given individually or by combining them together into one shot. People get the same protection with fewer shots, compared with individual vaccines given separately. Fewer shots means less pain and stress for the people, especially for infants and children. For example, infants and children may only get one shot to protect him from three or even five diseases, instead of three or five individual shots. Diphtheria, tetanus, and pertussis (DTP) vaccine and measles, mumps and rubella (MMR) vaccine are two successful combination vaccines [21]. Also, combining vaccines make more infants and children get recommended vaccinations on schedule. Because scientists are developing more combination vaccines against more diseases, combination vaccines may become more common in the near future.

4.3. Development of multiple administration routes

Most of the vaccines are given by injection such as intramuscular (IM), subcutaneous (SC), and intradermal (ID) injection. Additionally, mouths and nostrils are two successful alternative routes for administration. For example, Sabin vaccine (OPV) and FluMist® are given by oral administration and intranasal spray, respectively. These two methods are more effective, inexpensive, painless, and convenient than injection. Microparticles introduced by biotechnologies have made it possible to have an inactive *Vibrio cholera* whole-cell vaccine that changes its administration route from injection to oral administration in mice [22]. Furthermore, more methods of administering vaccines through biotechnologies are being developed including patches, aerosol inhalation, microneedles, and even eating of genetically modified organisms (GMO).

4.4. Development of synthetic vaccines

Synthetic vaccines are composed mainly of synthetic peptides, polysaccharides, or antigens. They are usually considered to be safer than vaccines from bacterial cultures, because they are developed by reconstructing the outside structure of a microbe, which helps to prevent vaccine resistance. Diphtheria toxoid is the first synthetic vaccine which was created in 1982. Creating vaccines synthetically can expedite a specific vaccine production [23]. This is particularly important in the outbreak of a pandemic disease.

4.5. Development of vaccines for both innate and adaptive immunity

Conventional vaccines only induce adaptive immunity, but vaccines are being designed to stimulate both innate and adaptive immune responses. This can be accomplished by the addition of an appropriate adjuvant such as CpG oligonucleotides [24].

4.6. Development of vaccines for preventing noninfectious diseases

Conventional vaccines are only used to prevent infectious diseases in which active immunization is largely confined to infectious diseases. However, vaccines are being developed to prevent many noninfectious human diseases such as cancer, type I diabetes mellitus (T1DM),

Alzheimer disease and drug addiction, etc. Mostly efforts are being directed against cancers. It has been very successful in reducing the incidence of hepatoma and cervical cancer using of HBV and HPV vaccines for preventing virus infection. Several types of preventive cancer vaccines are being tried such as antigen vaccines, tumor cell vaccines, dendritic vaccines, DNA vaccines, and viral vector vaccines [25]. Tolerization to autoantigens is being attempted in T1DM; the administration of diabetes-specific autoantigens can elicit tolerance, which can prevent the destruction of β-cells [26]. Alzheimer disease may be controlled by immunization against amyloid [27]. It is known that drug addictions (e.g. cocaine) may be controllable by inducing antibodies that rapidly remove the drugs from the body [28]. Recent studies further reveal that the activation of Toll-like receptor 9 (TLR9) can improve the function of cocaine vaccines in the presence of TLR5 activation [29].

4.7. Development of vaccines for therapy

Vaccines are conventionally prophylactic, but vaccines are being developed to treat chronic virus infection and cancer.

(1) Chronic virus infection: The induction of cellular immune response can suppress chronic virus infections such as HBV, hepatitis C virus (HCV), human immunodeficiency virus (HIV), and HPV [30].

(2) Cancer: Some cancers are difficult to treat by conventional methods such as surgery, radiation, chemotherapy, and target therapy, but can be controlled by the immune responses triggered by cancer vaccines. However, the development of these therapeutic vaccines is extremely challenging. Fortunately, expanded studies and knowledge regarding the mechanisms how cancer cells escape the immune system may develop new means in modulating the immune responses to cancer; thus, potentially enhancing the effectiveness of therapeutic cancer vaccines.

4.8. Development of vaccines for bioterrorism

Bioterrorist attack is unpleasant and rare, but it may happen unexpectedly and often leads to serious events. It is needed to develop vaccines to defend against bioterrorism agents such as anthrax, plague, smallpox, and even severe acute respiratory syndromes (SARS). Such vaccines must provide protection against pathogens that might enter the body by a variety of routes including the oral and respiratory tract. They should be given by noninvasive routes and able to induce protective immunity rapidly. The design of improved vaccines is likely to rely on the genome information of bioterrorism agents that have either completed or have almost completed sequencing [31].

5. Discussion

The development of powerful biotechnological tools applied to genome-based approaches has virtually revolutionized vaccine development. The information of genome provides a list of all the potential proteins from which it is possible for scientists to select some antigens or antigenic materials that are likely to be more effective vaccines [25]. Even if biotechnologies render many benefits for vaccine development, they are not always advantageous. The disadvantages include limited immunization to antigens, risk of affecting genes controlling cell growth, possibility of inducing antibody production against DNA, possibility of tolerance to the antigen produced, and potential for atypical processing of microbial proteins. In addition, it is a critical issue to formulate and deliver these vaccines appropriately to improve vaccine quality and expand their clinical application.

Vaccines dramatically reduce the incidence of serious infectious diseases and allow life expectancy of people to gradually increase. The persistent outbreak of many infectious diseases has decreased through vaccination; however, the burden of noninfectious diseases such as cancers, cardiovascular diseases, and diabetes mellitus has increased. This transformation of disease burden has indicated that the need for vaccines to treat or prevent noninfectious diseases is urgent. Both infectious and noninfectious diseases are now within the realm of vaccinology through the development of biotechnologies. Noninfectious disease vaccines also can be made by biotechnologies, but their target is human normal cells or abnormal cells, rather than pathogens or pathogen-infected cells. These vaccines present an interesting challenge for approving and evaluating under the same framework as traditional vaccines or that of other biologics, though they work by modulating the human immune system as traditional vaccines. Noninfectious disease vaccines have raised the question of whether the term "vaccine" is appropriate and some regulatory implications for this new category of drugs.

Despite vaccine development is rapid and clinical application is significantly expanded by biotechnologies, some infections, including HIV, HCV, SARS, MERS, Ebola virus, cytomegalovirus, and Zika virus, are under research and there are no effective vaccines available yet. Many vaccine candidates for these infections had been developed, but none had been approved for use in humans. The major difficulty for their clinical application is the lack of human clinical trials, the data insufficiency of for vaccine effectiveness, and the concern of vaccine safety. More funding, time, and research are needed for developing vaccines against recent emerging diseases such as MERS, Ebola virus, Zika virus infections, etc.

The perspectives for controlling diseases by vaccination are very promising along with the advancement of biotechnologies, but several problems are still hard to solve. First, vaccine supply is not sufficient even in the highly-developed countries, shortage of vaccines may occur due to regulatory pressures on production and the lack of qualified manufacturers. In the case of emergency, such as an influenza pandemic, it is difficult to estimate the demand of vaccine to satisfy the developing countries. Second, new vaccine discovery is very expensive and most of the manufacturers which do R&D have to pay the cost, but its revenue is limited. Some manufacturers may change their focusing products from vaccines to other medicinal products such as cell therapy products, gene therapy products, nanomedicines, and other products. Third, the requirement for vaccine safety is increasing, the evaluation of risk and benefit ratios become very crucial for the implementation of a vaccination program. But zero risk is almost impossible. It is quite difficult and controversial to obtain a balance between the need of public health and the regulatory impulse which guard against rare and theoretical risks.

6. Conclusion

Vaccination is the best approach to prevent infectious diseases. Vaccination is able to reduce the rates of mortality and morbidity from infection and results in herd immunity when some population has been vaccinated in some areas. Through vaccines distribution, some diseases are globally eradicated such as smallpox; some diseases are significantly controlled in much of the world such as polio, measles, and tetanus. However, there are many diseases uncontrolled yet by vaccination, and new diseases certainly appear through evolution, mutation, gene recombination, interspecies transfer, and environmental changes. Fortunately, we have many technologies to produce more novel vaccines to protect us. The previous studies have allowed us to understand the microbial pathogenesis and host immune responses which are correlated to the control of diseases by vaccination. Biotechnologies make it possible to further improve the quality of vaccines and expand the clinical application of vaccines significantly. More and more novel vaccine products based on biotechnologies are approved in the market around the world. Despite the great advances in biotechnologies, the perfect vaccine has not yet been developed. This vaccine would be temperature insensitive, multivalent and induce specific immunity against the protective antigens, would prevent and treat both diseases and possibly infections, would have long-term immunity without booster doses, free of adverse reactions, and administered without needles and the help of trained health workers. It is expectable to have such effective, cheap, and convenient vaccines for disease prevention and therapy provided that we endeavor to overcome the challenges in the production, distribution, and regulation of vaccines through biotechnologies.

Author details

Yuan-Chuan Chen[1], Hwei-Fang Cheng[1], Yi-Chen Yang[1] and Ming-Kung Yeh[2]*

*Address all correspondence to: mkyeh2004@gmail.com

1 Food and Drug Administration, Ministry of Health and Welfare, Taipei, Taiwan

2 School of Pharmacy, National Defense Medical Center, Taipei, Taiwan

References

[1] Chen YC, Cheng WF, Yang YC, Yeh MK. Nanotechnologies applied in biomedical vaccines. In: Stanciu SG, editor. Micro and Nanotechnologies for Biotechnology. Croatia: Intech; 2016. pp. 85-105. DOI: org/10.5772/63453

[2] Alessandro S, Rino R. Review: Reverse vaccinology: Developing vaccines in the era of genomics. Immunity. 2010;**33**(4):530-541. DOI: 10.1016/j.immuni.2010.09.017

[3] Delany I, Rappuoli R, Seib KL. Vaccines, reverse vaccinology, and bacterial pathogenesis. Cold Spring Harbor Perspectives Medicine. 2013;**3**(5):a012476. DOI: 10.1101/cshperspect.a012476

[4] Li D, von Schaewen M, Wang X, Tao W, Zhang Y, Li L, Heller B, Hrebikova G, Deng Q, Ploss A, Zhong J, Huang Z. Altered glycosylation patterns increase immunogenicity of a subunit hepatitis C virus vaccine, inducing neutralizing antibodies which confer protection in mice. Journal of Virology. 2016;**90**(23):10486-10498. DOI: 10.1128/JVI.01462-16

[5] Hansson M, Nygren PA, Stahl S. Design and production of recombinant subunit vaccines. Applied Biochemistry and Biotechnology. 2000;**32**(Pt 2):95-107. DOI: 10.1042/BA20000034

[6] Cox MM. Recombinant protein vaccines produced in insect cells. Vaccine. 2012;**30**(10): 1759-1766. DOI: 10.1016/j.vaccine.2012.01.016

[7] Cockrell AS, Baric RS. An effective DNA vaccine platform for Middle East respiratory syndrome coronavirus. Annals Translational Medicine. 2016;**4**(24):499. DOI: 10.21037/atm.2016.11.40

[8] Ferraro B, Morrow MP, Hutnick NA, Shin TH, Lucke CE, Weiner DB. Clinical applications of DNA vaccines: Current progress. Clinical Infectious Diseases. 2011;**53**(3):296-302. DOI: 10.1093/cid/cir334

[9] Sahin U,Karikó K, Türeci Ö. mRNA-based therapeutics- developing a new class of drugs. Nature Reviews Drug Discovery. 2014;**13**:759-780. DOI: 10.1038/nrd4278

[10] Schlake T, Thess A, Fotin-Mleczek M, Kallen KJ. Developing mRNA-vaccine technologies. RNA Biology. 2012;**9**(11):1319-1330. DOI: 10.4161/rna.22269

[11] Chang M-H, Chen C-J, Lai M-S, Hsu H-M, Wu T-C, Kong M-S, Liang D-C, Shau W-Y, Chen D-S. Universal Hepatitis B vaccination in Taiwan and the incidence of hepatocellular carcinoma in children. New England Journal of Medicine. 1997;**336**(26):1855-1859. DOI: 10.1056/NEJM199706263362602, DOI:10.1056%2FNEJM199706263362602

[12] Ma L, Wang X, Bi X, Yang J, Shi B, He X, Ma R, Ma Q, Yao X. Characteristics peripheral blood IgG and IgM heavy chain complementarity determining region 3 repertoire before and after immunization with recombinant HBV vaccine. PLoS One. 2017;**12**(1):e0170479. DOI: 10.1371/journal.pone.0170479

[13] McCarthy M. Project seeks to "fast track" rotavirus vaccine. Lancet. 2003;**361**(9357):582. DOI: 10.1016/S0140-6736(03)12549-4 DOI: 10.1016%2FS0140-6736%2803%2912549-4

[14] Gautam R, Mijatovic-Rustempasic S, Esona MD, Tam KI, Quaye O, Bowen MD. One-step multiplex real-time RT-PCR assay for detecting and genotyping wild-type group A rotavirus strains and vaccine strains (Rotarix® and RotaTeq®) in stool samples. Peer Journal. 2016;**4**:e1560. DOI: 10.7717/peerj.1560

[15] Monie A, Hung CF, Roden R, Wu TC. Cervarix™: A vaccine for the prevention of HPV 16, 18-associated cervical cancer. Biologics. 2008;**2**(1):107-113. Available from: http://www.ncbi.nlm.nih.gov/pmc/articles/PMC2727782/pdf/btt-2-107.pdf

[16] Kash N, Lee MA, Kollipara R, Downing C, Guidry J, Tyring SK. Safety and efficacy data on vaccines and immunization to human papillomavirus. Journal of Clinical Medicine Research. 2015;4(4):614-633. DOI: 10.3390/jcm4040614. Review

[17] Ferguson NM, Rodríguez-Barraquer I, Dorigatti I, Mier-y-Teran-Romero L, Laydon DJ, Cummings DAT. Benefits and risks of the Sanofi-Pasteur dengue vaccine: Modeling Optimal Deployment. Science. 2016;**353**(6303):1033-1036. DOI: 10.1126/science.aaf9590

[18] Aguiar M, Stollenwerk N, Halstead SB. The Impact of the newly licensed dengue vaccine in endemic countries. PLoS Neglected Tropical Diseases. 2016;**10**(12):e0005179. DOI: 10.1371/journal.pntd.0005179

[19] Scott LJ. Tetravalent dengue vaccine: A review in the prevention of dengue disease. Drugs. 2016;**76**(13):1301-1312. DOI: 10.1007/s40265-016-0626-8

[20] Serruto D, Adu-Bobie J, Capecchi B, Rappuoli R, Pizza M, Masignani V. Biotechnology and vaccines: application of functional genomics to *Neisseria meningitidis* and other bacterial pathogens. Journal of Biotechnology. 2004;**113**(1-3):15-32. DOI: 10.1016/j.jbiotec.2004.03.024

[21] Skibinski DA, Baudner BC, Singh M, O'Hagan DT. Combination vaccines. Journal of Global Infectious Diseases. 2011;**3**(1):63-72. DOI: 10.4103/0974-777X.77298, DOI:10.4103%2F0974-777X.77298#pmc_ext

[22] Yeh MK, Chiang CH. Inactive Vibro cholera whole-cell vaccine-loaded biodegradable microparticles: In vitro release and oral vaccination. Journal of Microencapsulation. 2004;**21**(1):91-106. DOI: 10.1080/02652040310001619794

[23] Young S. Synthetic Biology Could Speed Flu Vaccine Production. MIT Technology Review. 2013. Available from: http://www.technologyreview.com/news/514661/synthetic-biology-could-speed-flu-vaccine-production/

[24] Klinman DM. Immunotherapeutic uses of CpG oligodeoxynucleotides. Nature Reviews Immunology. 2004;**4**(4):249-258. DOI: 10.1038/nri1329

[25] Mohammed S, Bakshi N, Chaudri N, Akhter J, Akhtar M. Cancer vaccines: Past, Present, and Future. Advances in Anatomic Pathology. 2016;**23**(3):180-191. DOI: 10.1097/PAP.0000000000000116

[26] Orban T, Kis JT. Prevention of Type 1 diabetes mellitus using a novel vaccine. Therapeutic Advances in Endocrinology and Metabolism. 2011;**2**(1):9-16. DOI: 10.1177/2042018810390546 DOI:10.1177%2F2042018810390546#pmc_ext

[27] Rygiel K, Novel strategies for Alzheimer's disease treatment: An overview of anti-amyloid beta monoclonal antibodies. Indian Journal of Pharmacology. 2016;**48**(6):629-636. DOI: 10.4103/0253-7613.194867

[28] Kantak KM, Collins SL, Lipman EG, Bond J, Giovanoni K, Fox BS. Evaluation of anti-cocaine antibodies and a cocaine vaccine in a rat self-administration model. Psychopharmacology (Berl). 2000;**148**(3):251-262. doi.org/10.1007/s002130050049

[29] Kimishima A, Wenthur CJ, Eubanks LM, Sato S, Janda KD. Cocaine vaccine development: Evaluation of carrier and adjuvant combinations that activate multiple Toll-Like receptors. Molecular Pharmaceutics. 2016;**13**(11):3884-3890. DOI: 10.1021/acs.molpharmaceut.6b00682

[30] Plotkin SA. Vaccines: Past, present and future. Nature Medicine. 2005;**11**(4 Suppl):S5-S11. DOI: 10.1038/nm1209

[31] Titball RW, Williamson ED. Vaccine development for potential bioterrorism agents. Current Drug Targets Infectious Disorders. 2003;**3**(3):255-262. doi.org/10.2174/1568005033481097

Section 5

Engineering Effective Vaccines

Chapter 6

The Use of Planar Electromagnetic Fields in Effective Vaccine Design

Adrián Cortés, Jonathan Coral, Colin McLachlan and
Ricardo Benítez

Additional information is available at the end of the chapter

http://dx.doi.org/10.5772/intechopen.69546

Abstract

Vaccines have not yet been able to address the combination of three major obstacles: molecular coupling failure between peptide and human leukocyte antigen protein (HLA-II) molecule, failure to activate T-cells, and the molecular polymorphism displayed by all pathogens. Planar electromagnetic fields found in protein systems may play a role in all three problems. These amino acid planes are universal, selective in nature, and able to generate long distance attraction toward their corresponding ligand. We propose three molecular mechanisms through which to engineer molecular pattern interaction toward the intelligent design of more effective vaccines.

Keywords: vaccine design, PECC, HLA-II binding affinity, T-cell activation, molecular polymorphism

1. Introduction

Many different technologies have been developed to design different types of vaccines—biological, synthetic, genetically engineered, naked DNA and vector—and in spite of these efforts, major problems remain to be solved, preventing effective vaccines being obtained for pathogens such as HIV and malaria.

Three obstacles for current vaccines relate to the difficulty in coupling class II human leukocyte antigen proteins (HLA-II), in activating T-helper cells, and the molecular polymorphism of the pathogens.

Our search for solutions to these obstacles led to a series of significant findings, fundamental to biochemistry, and relating to: the discovery of the mechanism of molecular coupling between peptides and HLA-II molecules; identification of the mechanism for the activation of T-cell receptor molecules; a solution to molecular polymorphism in pathogens.

2. Molecular coupling between peptides and HLA-II molecules

In the activation of immune responses, HLA-II molecules are responsible for presenting peptide antigens to T-helper cells [1, 2] to activate the cascade that accompanies this response. The coupling of HLA-II molecules with peptide antigens is therefore critical for vaccine design [3, 4] because it is necessary to induce immune memory.

All the subtypes of HLA-II molecules (DR, DP and DQ) are highly polymorphic [1, 5]. The high polymorphism of these molecules represents one of the greatest difficulties in vaccine development [2–4], as HLA-II/peptide coupling is restricted by this polymorphism.

2.1. Planar electromagnetic fields in HLA-II molecules may explain coupling with foreign peptides

Following a review of HLA-II molecules from the National Center for Biotechnology Information (NCBI) database, the constant positions of fully conserved residues in HLA-II α and β chains were identified. The positions are recorded in **Table 1**.

These positions were then located within a three-dimensional protein crystallography structure provided by the protein data bank (PDB) and examined using bioinformatic tools, whereupon geometric patterns emerged.

Fully conserved residues	Residues in the HLA-II molecules, in the α and β chains						Aromatic residue in the plane (3O6F)
	DP (3LQZ)[a]		DQ (1UVQ)		DR (1DLH)		
	α	β	α	β	α	β	
Cys (C)	107	15, 115, 171	110	15, 117, 173	107	117, 173	Phe - 151
Gly (G)	100, 131	149, 166	103, 134	151, 168	131	151, 168	Tyr - 150
Leu (L)	105, 151	113, 159	108, 154	115, 161	105, 151	115, 161	Phe - 184
Asn (N)	103	31, 60, 132, 148	106	33, 62, 134, 150	103	134, 150	Phe - 151
Pro (P)	102, 114, 115, 155	95, 122, 163	105, 117, 118, 158	97, 124, 165	102, 114, 115, 155	97, 124, 165	Phe - 137
Thr (T)	-	152, 170	-	154, 172	-	154, 172	Phe - 184
Val (V)	91	97, 117, 173	94	99, 119, 175	91, 128	99, 119, 175	Phe - 151
Trp (W)	121	129, 151, 186	124	131, 153, 188	121	131, 153, 188	Trp - 182
Tyr (Y)	150	121, 169	153	123, 171	150	123, 171	Tyr - 152

Note: [a]PDB ID are shown in parenthesis.

Table 1. Fully conserved residues of HLA-II in sequences and structures.

These molecular patterns were found in all three types of HLA-II (DR, DP and DQ). They comprise fully conserved amino acid residues arranged in a planar configuration. **Figure 1** illustrates the spatial arrangements for the amino acid residues Gly (**Figure 1a** and **b**) and Trp (**Figure 1c** and **d**).

The patterns were found to feature the conditions required to generate planar electromagnetic fields. These fields are known as planar electromagnetic fields of Cortés-Coral (PECC). PECC fields are produced by groups of invariant and fully conserved amino acids from a single chemical species (this conservation is simultaneous both in sequence and in space). There will thus, for example, be glycine planes (PECC-Gly), proline planes (PECC-Pro), leucine planes (PECC-Leu), etc. Importantly, each PECC field is generated in a single direction.

The question may arise as to how the electromagnetic field is generated. Essential to the explanation is the fact that each plane was found to possess an aromatic amino acid (e.g., Phe, Tyr, Trp) always located in a well-defined position within that plane. An aromatic amino acid has electric charges in motion (electrons). These electrons generate the electromagnetic signals that are able to act over long molecular distances, i.e., at long range. The HLA-II/peptide coupling mechanism has not been able to be explained satisfactorily by the already known intermolecular forces (Van der Waals, hydrogen bonding and ionic forces) because they act only at short range; in the case of ionic forces [6], for example, the range of

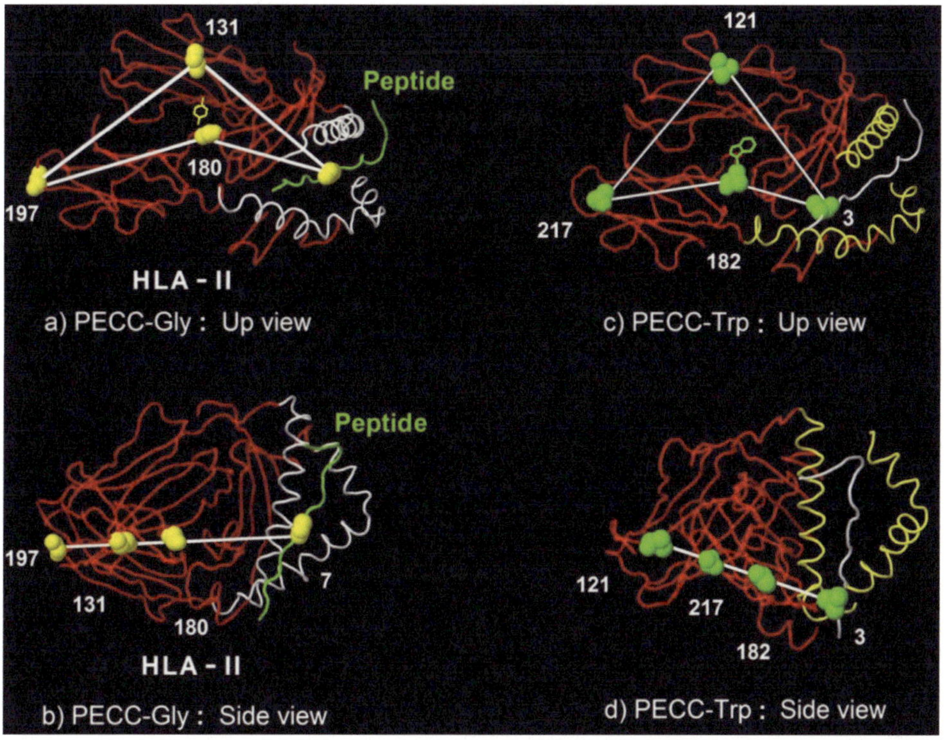

Figure 1. Spatial positions of fully conserved glycine and tryptophan residues in HLA-II DR (Images taken from Jmol 12.0, reproduced with permission of IVSI).

action is only about 2 nm [7]. It follows, therefore, that no classical concept is able to explain the long-range molecular interactions that occur between protein molecules. Further, in three-dimensional analysis of proteins and their ligands, it can be seen that the couplings do not have a well-defined or selective spatial and electrostatic complementarity, as proposed by the "key-lock" model [8, 9]. There is evidence, meanwhile, that biological processes can be induced or modulated by electromagnetic fields of characteristic frequencies, as with light in photosynthetic systems [10] or with the increase in the catalytic activity of some enzymes on being irradiated with electromagnetic fields [11, 12]. Research carried out by the School of Electrical and Computer Engineering of the RMIT University in Melbourne (Australia) shows that proteins emit and absorb electromagnetic radiation of very precise frequencies, different for each protein [8].

PECC fields, as we have seen by their planar nature, act in a single and specific direction. They are also able to act over long distances. They are therefore capable of explaining the following phenomena intrinsic to receptor-ligand coupling:

- the *directional nature* of the attraction/coupling;
- the *selectivity* required to target the correct ligand;
- the extremely *short time* period to encounter the ligand;
- and the *long distance* across which the attraction must take place.

In this context, given the three-dimensional arrangement of each PECC based on the positions of its component residues in the protein structure, each PECC field of HLA-II was projected in the direction of its plane toward the HLA-II groove pockets. Specific positions on the groove were thus associated with the PECC projections.

When a foreign peptide is in the coupled position, each of the positions identified is found to contain a residue of exactly the same species as the PECC projected there; where a PECC-Gly is projected onto the groove, a glycine residue is encountered in the coupled foreign peptide. Similarly, for a PECC-Leu projection, a leucine residue is found at that position. The PECC projections were thus able to predict residues and their positions in the groove.

The universal Class II-associated invariant chain peptide (CLIP), known for its binding affinity, was further found to have five PECC projection matches. When CLIP was modified so that it contained an additional PECC projection, its binding affinity was enhanced, suggesting that PECC fields favor the attraction of their respective residue in a peptide [13, 14].

Using PECC projections toward the groove of HLA-II molecules, a universal coupling sequence was found to be present in all HLA-II types. This is presented in **Table 2**. Note that more than one PECC may be projected toward some positions, as shown for position 1, where PECC-Trp, PECC-Tyr and PECC-Val are present.

Considering this finding further, a pattern of universal coupling was identified in all types and subtypes of histocompatibility molecule, thus permitting the design of peptide-vaccines with a capacity to couple with any polymorphic form presented by HLA-II molecules [13].

PECC position in groove of HLA-II											
–1	1	2	3	4	5	6	7	8	9	10	11
L	W	P	P	W	W	P	L	L	N	P	P
V	Y	C			T		G	P		N	
	V				G		P				

Table 2. PECC fields projected toward different positions of the HLA-II anchoring groove.

The application of this new finding made it possible to design peptides with better peptide/HLA-II coupling values than those generated by the universal coupling peptide CLIP [13, 14].

Selection and attraction between HLA-II molecules and antigen peptides in this way would therefore be nonrandom, resulting in an effective and rapid coupling mechanism, as is clearly required in the immune response. Thus, PECC fields project outwardly from the HLA-II molecule in order to select, attract, and couple specific peptide sequences (**Figure 2**).

Application of the principles of this selective and attractive force could permit the design in future of vaccine-peptides with a universal high binding affinity to HLA-II molecules. The findings would further allow new avenues to be explored involving other protein systems, including HLA-I and T-cell receptors (TCRs), necessary for understanding mechanisms of immune activation, as well as opening up possibilities for the wider study of protein receptor-ligand systems.

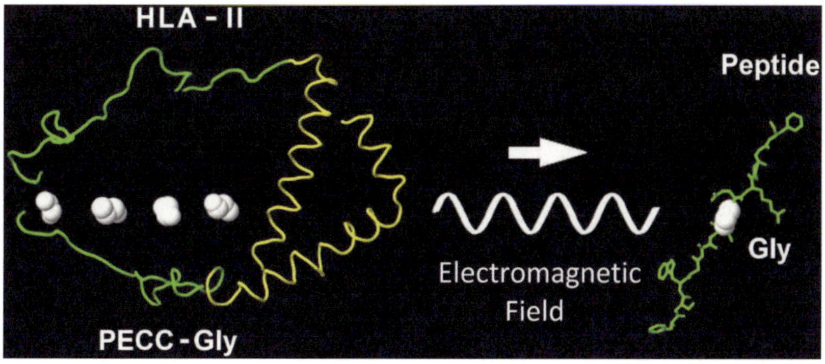

Figure 2. PECC-Gly selective, attractive force, exerted toward Gly residue in peptide (Images taken from Jmol 12.0, reproduced with permission of IVSI).

3. Activation of T-helper cells

T-cell receptors (TCRs) are molecules found on the surface of T-helper cells that are responsible for recognizing antigens bound to HLA-II molecules. This coupling is very important for immune memory, whenever activation of the TCRs occurs. TCR activation is provoked on recognition of certain foreign antigens (T-epitopes) and is crucial to the functioning of vaccines [15, 16]. Thus, all vaccines require T-epitopes in their protein composition, acting as TCR activators. However, the mechanisms known to induce activation are not clearly understood [17]. Greater comprehension in this regard could enable the design of vaccine-peptides capable of inducing immunological memory in B and T cell lines.

A number of authors refer to the TCR as a "mechanosensor" that converts mechanical energy into biochemical signals on coupling with the antigen, whereupon transduction of the signal is induced [18, 19]. However, this mechanistic explanation is not sufficient to understand the internalization of the message induced by the ligand, since a mechanism of this type requires too much energy to induce a signal that travels all the way from the point of coupling with the ligand to the intracellular domain. This is because a mechanical signal induces multiple aimless movements, raising the entropy of the system, and dispersing the energy [20]. Moreover, such an activation mechanism would not be sufficiently specific and would lack the selectivity necessary to differentiate between the body's own antigens and foreign ones.

Researchers at the IVSI institute put forward an explanation for understanding the molecular mechanisms of activation and transduction in the TCRs, based on the concept of PECC. The fully conserved residues found in the TCR molecules are shown in **Table 3**. These residues form a PECC system responsible for transmitting the signal of the antigen from its point of contact to the interior of the cell. This type of field was termed PECC-ionic, or PECC-i [21]. Only the alpha (α) chain of the TCR showed fully conserved residues that form part of the PECC-i. No such residues were evident in the beta (β) chain.

From physical analysis of a PECC-i, it may be inferred that all of its residues are mutually interlinked by a single electromagnetic field. This field would ensure that the residues behave in a synchronized manner. As a result, the action applied at one point (amino acid) of the PECC-i is replicated at all the other points, enabling signals to be sent from the point of contact with the ligand to the intracellular domain of the receptor [21], as shown in **Figure 3**. In **Figure 3a–c**, all the highly conserved residues of the free TCRs are seen to be in a dissociated state, while in **Figure 3d**, in which the molecule is coupled with the peptide, these same residues are paired. This shows that the coupling of opposite charges between the TCR and the peptide induces the additional formation of new pairings inside the planar system. The mechanism proposed by the authors to explain the molecular transduction of signals was named "molecular transduction by PECC-ionic" (TM-PECC–i, from the Spanish acronym) [21].

PDB	1FYT	4GKZ	3QEU	3QH3
Residues of human TCRs[a]	D135	D133	D128	D129
	K136	K134	K129	K130
	K184	K182	K177	K178
	D 186	D184	D179	D180

Note:[a] Residues in the α–chain of the TCR molecule.

Table 3. Fully conserved residues in human TCR molecules that form PECC planes. Such residues occupy equivalent spatial positions in all TCRs.

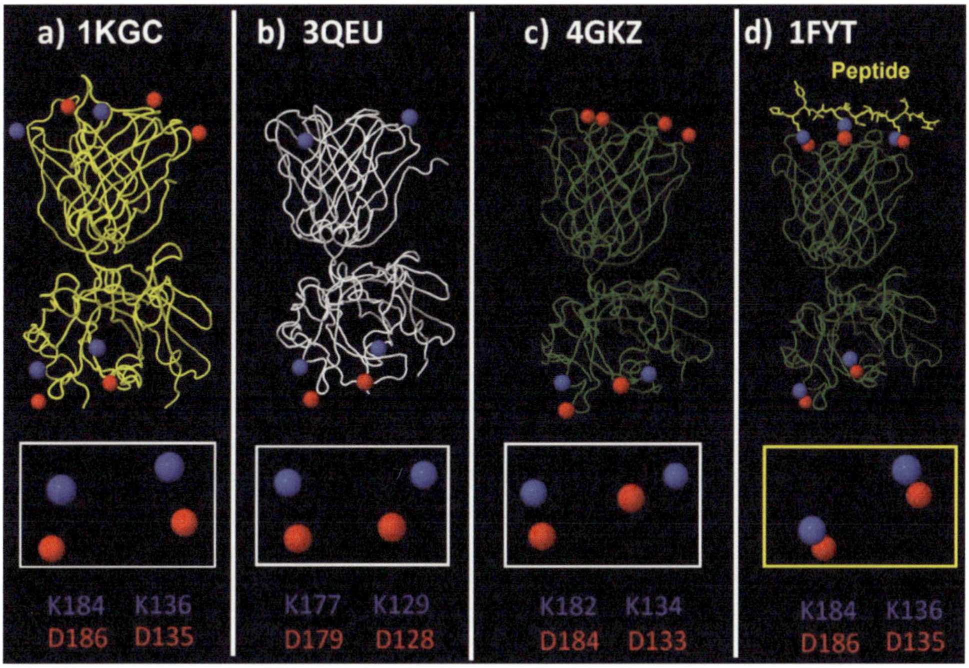

Figure 3. TCR molecules in free states (a–c) and coupled (d), showing positive and negative electrical residues as stylized spheres. The highly conserved residues are highlighted in the boxes below each figure. (Image records taken from Jmol, reproduced with permission of IVSI) [21].

4. Molecular polymorphism of pathogens

Molecular polymorphism is a mechanism that pathogenic agents employ to evade host immune responses. None of the current vaccines has managed to overcome this problem, which is why vaccination booster doses require to be applied anew each year, as in the case of influenza. The HIV virus and the malarial parasite are highly polymorphic pathogens that change their molecular sequences every time they replicate.

The IVSI Institute was the first research group in the world to find a solution to the molecular polymorphism of pathogens. The authors found that the molecular polymorphism of a pathogen is not random but rather ruled by an underlying order that allows the protein to retain its functionality while evading repeated attack by the immune system. By re-examining the molecular cell-pathogen coupling receptors in the new light of PECC fields, a solution to molecular polymorphism in pathogens was found.

The method developed by our researchers to solve the problem of the polymorphism of the virus is analogous to what happens with the bedroom door-key system in a 200-room hotel: each guest will have a key to open his/her own room, so that 200 keys will be needed to open all of the rooms. The concierge, however, is not required to carry around 200 keys. He will have a single key, or master key, to be able to open every door. Likewise, our methodology enabled us to identify the the master key used by the virus in order to couple *always with the same receptor*, despite its high molecular polymorphism, using solid state physics tools. Using these tools together with the PECC system raises the possibility of designing effective vaccines against the polymorphic pathogen.

5. Conclusions

A novel methodology is proposed by the authors for the design of effective vaccines, based on planar molecular patterns found in proteins. These patterns were discovered in fully conserved residues of HLA-II and TCR molecules. According to the authors, these patterns generate planar electromagnetic fields, given the name PECC fields. These direct the coupling of peptides with HLA-II molecules and the activation of the TCRs in T-cells. The function of these PECC fields is to select and attract antigen-peptides for subsequent coupling with HLA-II molecules. A further type of PECC, known as PECC-ionic, is responsible for interiorizing the signal of TCR-antigen coupling to activate the T-helper cells. Moreover, the PECC concept enabled the authors to solve the problem of molecular polymorphism of pathogens, finding an underlying order in the apparent random chaos of polymorphism.

Acknowledgements

The authors express their gratitude to the Synthetic Vaccines, Antisera and New Drugs Research Institute (IVSI) Colombia for providing the infrastructure and funding for developing the model. We are also grateful to the University of Cauca for continuing support.

Author details

Adrián Cortés[1], Jonathan Coral[1], Colin McLachlan[1] and Ricardo Benítez[2]*

*Address all correspondence to: rbenitez@unicauca.edu.co

1 Department of Molecular Physics, Synthetic Vaccine and New Drug Research Institute, IVSI, Popayán, Colombia

2 Department of Chemistry, Natural Product Chemistry Research Group, University of Cauca, Popayán, Colombia

References

[1] Reinherz EL, Tan K, Tang L, Kern P, Liu J-h, Xiong Y, et al. The crystal structure of a T cell receptor in complex with peptide and MHC class II. Science. 1999;**286**:1913-1921

[2] Mushtaq K, Chodisetti SB, Rai PK, Maurya SK, Amir M, Sheikh JA, et al. Decision-making critical amino acids: Role in designing peptide vaccines for eliciting Th1 and Th2 immune response. Amino acids. 2014;**46**:1265-1274

[3] Desai DV, Kulkarni-Kale U. T-cell Epitope Prediction Methods: An Overview. Immunoinformatics. Springer; 2014. pp. 333-364

[4] Ribeiro SP, Rosa DS, Fonseca SG, Mairena EC, Postól E, Oliveira SC, et al. A vaccine encoding conserved promiscuous HIV CD4 epitopes induces broad T cell responses in mice transgenic to multiple common HLA class II molecules. PLoS One. 2010;**5**: e11072

[5] Wang M, Claesson MH. Classification of Human Leukocyte Antigen (HLA) Supertypes. Immunoinformatics. Springer; 2014. pp. 309-317

[6] Kumar S, Nussinov R. Close-range electrostatic interactions in proteins. ChemBioChem. 2002;**3**:604-617

[7] Beretta S, Chirico G, Baldini G. Short-range interactions of globular proteins at high ionic strengths. Macromolecules. 2000;**33**:8663-8670

[8] Ćosić I, Pirogova E, Vojisavljević V, Fang Q. Electromagnetic properties of biomolecules. FME Transactions. 2006;**34**:71-80

[9] Pirogova E, Cosic I, Vojisavljevic V. Biological Effects of Electromagnetic Radiation. INTECH Open Access Publisher; 2009

[10] Brédas J-L, Sargent EH, Scholes GD. Photovoltaic concepts inspired by coherence effects in photosynthetic systems. Nature Materials. 2017;**16**:35-44

[11] Vojisavljevic V, Pirogova E, Cosic I, editors. Influence of electromagnetic radiation on enzyme kinetics. Engineering in Medicine and Biology Society, 2007 EMBS 2007 29th Annual International Conference of the IEEE. IEEE; 2007

[12] Vojisavljevic V, Pirogova E, Cosic I, editors. Review of studies on modulating enzyme activity by low intensity electromagnetic radiation. Engineering in Medicine and Biology Society (EMBC), 2010 Annual International Conference of the IEEE. IEEE; 2010

[13] Cortes A, Coral J. Campos electromagneticos planares permiten explicar el acople entre peptidos y moleculas de HLA-II. Acta bioquímica clínica latinoamericana. 2015;**49**:221-228

[14] Cortés A, Coral J, Benítez Benítez R. Hallazgo de patrones para péptidos-vacuna con capacidad de acople universal en moléculas de HLA-II. Acta bioquímica clínica latinoamericana. 2013;**47**:541-549

[15] Sami M, Rizkallah PJ, Dunn S, Molloy P, Moysey R, Vuidepot A, et al. Crystal structures of high affinity human T-cell receptors bound to peptide major histocompatibility complex reveal native diagonal binding geometry. Protein Engineering Design and Selection. 2007;**20**:397-403

[16] Wang J-H, Reinherz EL. Revisiting the putative TCR Cα dimerization model through structural analysis. Frontiers in Immunology. 2013;**4**:16

[17] Adams JJ, Narayanan S, Liu B, Birnbaum ME, Kruse AC, Bowerman NA, et al. T cell receptor signaling is limited by docking geometry to peptide-major histocompatibility complex. Immunity. 2011;**35**:681-693

[18] Kim ST, Shin Y, Brazin K, Mallis RJ, Sun J, Wagner G, et al. TCR mechanobiology: Torques and tunable structures linked to early T cell signaling. Frontiers in Immunology. 2012;**3**:76

[19] Kim ST, Takeuchi K, Sun Z-YJ, Touma M, Castro CE, Fahmy A, et al. The $\alpha\beta$ T cell receptor is an anisotropic mechanosensor. Journal of Biological Chemistry. 2009;**284**:31028-31037

[20] Bischof M, Del Giudice E. Communication and the emergence of collective behavior in living organisms: A quantum approach. Molecular Biology International. 2013;**2013**

[21] Cortés A, Coral J, Benítez Benítez R, McLachlan C. Campos electromagnéticos planares permiten explicar transducción en receptores de células T. Acta bioquímica clínica latinoamericana. 2016;**50**:657-654

Chapter 7

The Impact of Bioinformatics on Vaccine Design and Development

Ribas-Aparicio Rosa María,
Castelán-Vega Juan Arturo, Jiménez-Alberto Alicia,
Monterrubio-López Gloria Paulina and
Aparicio-Ozores Gerardo

Additional information is available at the end of the chapter

http://dx.doi.org/10.5772/intechopen.69273

Abstract

Vaccines are the pharmaceutical products that offer the best cost-benefit ratio in the prevention or treatment of diseases. In that a vaccine is a pharmaceutical product, vaccine development and production are costly and it takes years for this to be accomplished. Several approaches have been applied to reduce the times and costs of vaccine development, mainly focusing on the selection of appropriate antigens or antigenic structures, carriers, and adjuvants. One of these approaches is the incorporation of bioinformatics methods and analyses into vaccine development. This chapter provides an overview of the application of bioinformatics strategies in vaccine design and development, supplying some successful examples of vaccines in which bioinformatics has furnished a cutting edge in their development. Reverse vaccinology, immunoinformatics, and structural vaccinology are described and addressed in the design and development of specific vaccines against infectious diseases caused by bacteria, viruses, and parasites. These include some emerging or re-emerging infectious diseases, as well as therapeutic vaccines to fight cancer, allergies, and substance abuse, which have been facilitated and improved by using bioinformatics tools or which are under development based on bioinformatics strategies.

Keywords: reverse vaccinology, immunoinformatics, structural vaccinology, computational strategies, vaccine

1. Introduction

The success of vaccination is reflected in its worldwide impact by improving human and veterinary health and life expectancy. It has been asserted that vaccination, as well as clean water, has had such a major effect on mortality reduction and population growth [1, 2]. In addition to the invaluable role of traditional vaccines to prevent diseases, the society has observed remarkable scientific and technological progress since the last century in the improvement of these vaccines and the generation of new ones. This has been possible by the fusion of computational technologies with the application of recombinant DNA technology, the fast growth of biological and genomic information in database banks, and the possibility of accelerated and massive sequencing of complete genomes [3–5]. This has aided in expanding the concept and application of vaccines beyond their traditional immunoprophylactic function of preventing infectious diseases, and also serving as therapeutic products capable of modifying the evolution of a disease and even cure it [3]. Vaccines are the pharmaceutical products that offer the best cost-benefit ratio in the prevention or treatment of diseases. In that it is a pharmaceutical product, a vaccine development and production are costly and it takes years for this to be accomplished. Several approaches have been applied to reduce the times and costs of their development, mainly focusing on the selection of appropriate antigens or antigenic structures, carriers, and adjuvants [6]. One of these approaches is the incorporation of bioinformatics methods and analyses into vaccine development. At present, there are many alternative strategies to design and develop effective and safe new-generation vaccines, based on bioinformatics approaches through reverse vaccinology, immunoinformatics, and structural vaccinology [7]. This chapter provides an overview of the application of bioinformatics strategies in vaccine design and development, supplying some successful examples of vaccines in which bioinformatics has furnished a cutting edge in their development.

2. Reverse vaccinology

Reverse vaccinology is a methodology that uses bioinformatics tools for the identification of structures from bacteria, virus, parasites, cancer cells, or allergens that could induce an immune response capable of protecting against a specific disease [7].

This approach possesses many advantages over traditional vaccinology: it reduces time and cost in vaccine development; refines the number of proteins to be studied, facilitating the selection process; can identify antigens present in small amounts or expressed only at certain stages, which would hinder or prevent their purification; and allows for the study of noncultivable or risky microorganisms [3]

An important requirement for utilizing this methodology is the availability of genomic information of the pathogen under study and, in some instances, even the human or animal cell genome must be known (i.e., DNA vaccines and therapeutic vaccines). Once the genome sequence is obtained, it is possible to identify all likely proteins that could be expressed. For this purpose, several software systems and programs identify all open reading frames (ORFs) that constitute the sequences expressing the majority of proteins [8–10].

The next step in reverse vaccinology is to determine several antigenic and physicochemical properties that have been associated with good antigens. These characteristics must be analyzed for each protein in the proteome under study, employing different bioinformatics approaches to select the protein(s) with the best properties for testing through *in vitro* and *in vivo* assays, in order to demonstrate its safety and immunogenicity. With the best vaccine candidates, different types of vaccines can be designed and developed, for example: subunit, recombinant, and nucleic acid vaccines [11].

The first application of reverse vaccinology was to study *Neisseria meningitidis* to obtain a new subunit vaccine based on the genome study of this microorganism by means of bioinformatics tools [12]. Thereafter, this technology has been used to study pathogenic agents including eukaryotic organisms and those involved in diseases transmitted by vectors [13], to design and obtain not only vaccines for humans but also for animals [5]. The majority of new vaccines against infectious diseases that have been developed with this technology are currently found in preclinical or clinical trial. However, it is important to mention that in some instances, the vaccine candidate obtained by this technology could fail as a good vaccine antigen, because it is identified based solely on computational probabilistic studies, and there are other factors that could interfere when this antigen is administered in a complete organism. In addition, vaccine candidates identified by this technology are restricted to proteins or lipoproteins, in that they are encoded in the genome. By reverse vaccinology, it is impossible to identify carbohydrate or lipid antigenic molecules [3, 14].

Some of the important properties to detect good vaccine candidates are described as follows:

2.1. Protein cellular localization

Proteins are localized in different parts of the cell: in the cytoplasm, the cell membrane, or they can be secreted out of the cell and become extracellular. Molecules localized on the cell membrane or extracellularly are better antigens because they are more exposed to host cells, specifically to those related to the immune system; thus, they have a greater probability of generating a protective response [15]. In addition to the software that can predict these characteristics, there are protein databases that generate information about protein subcellular localization, such as LOCATE, LocDB, and eSLDB.

2.2. Adhesin properties

In an infectious process, the first contact of the microorganism with the host cells is through adhesins. Molecules with adhesin properties are vaccine candidates [16]. The probability of identifying an adhesin is calculated based on the frequency of amino acids, dipeptides, or homopolymers present in the protein, and the physicochemical characteristics of each amino acid that constitutes a protein: acidic, basic, neutral, hydrophilic, or hydrophobic. There are programs that analyze all of these characteristics, comparing them with those of adhesins that have been previously proven experimentally [17].

2.3. Antigenicity

There are known sequences of antigens with good *in vivo* and *in vitro* immunologic inductions that are compared with each sequence of the proteome under study in order to search for similarities. In this case, it is probable that two proteins with similar sequences have comparable antigenic effects. Moreover, predictions of independent antigenicity alignment exist based on the physicochemical properties of amino acids [18].

2.4. Similarity

It is important to study the similarity between the sequences under study with molecules from the host that will receive the vaccine, as well as between the related etiological agents. Molecules with a high degree of similarity could generate two different effects: the first is undesirable because the antigen could cause autoimmune reactions; on the other hand, if the molecules are similar between other etiological agents, the vaccine could induce cross-protection [19]. In the case of a vaccine against cancer, it is important to select molecules present in cancer cells but absent in healthy cells. The similarity analysis can also be utilized to search for molecules with the same function, providing an idea of antigenicity and virulence [20]. It is important to predict these values because the main characteristic of a vaccine must be innocuous; in this way, if it is inferred that a protein can be antigenic but also toxic, the better course is not to use it.

2.5. Transmembrane helix

A transmembrane helix is a protein segment of 17–25 amino acids that conforms an α-helix structure that spans through the membrane cell. Most of the time, vaccine candidates are expressed in biological systems that are different from the original source; in that case, the three-dimensional (3D) structure of the protein could be changed or difficult to purify if it has a transmembrane helix, due to differences in membrane structure [21]. The low transmembrane helix number is a major characteristic for the selection of a vaccine candidate.

According to the etiology of the disease under study, protein cellular localization, adhesin properties, antigenicity, lack of homology with human proteins to avoid the induction of a potential autoimmune response, and low or null transmembrane helix structures are the main properties that should be identified. This can be addressed by utilizing several computer programs to analyze each of these properties and by bioinformatics tools for the screening and selection of vaccine candidates, according to their top feature values.

There are Websites and downloadable software that can be useful for a particular reverse vaccinology analysis, for example, NERVE, Vaxign, Jenner-predict server, and Vacceed. In some cases, the proteome-of-interest can be uploaded, and in others the organism in a specific database needed to be chosen; for this analysis, some characteristics about the agent and the host are required. In addition, there are databases with vaccine candidates already identified or with complete information about vaccines, for example VIOLIN and MycobacRV (**Table 1**).

Characteristic	Description	Software
Protein cellular localization	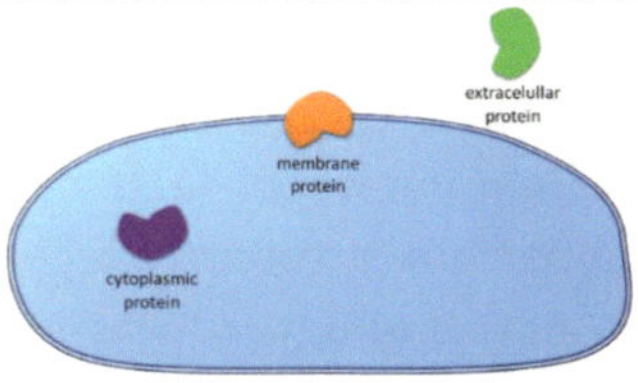	• Psortb • CELLO • TargetP • Cell-PLoc • LocDB • LocTree 2/3 • MultiLoc2
Adhesin properties	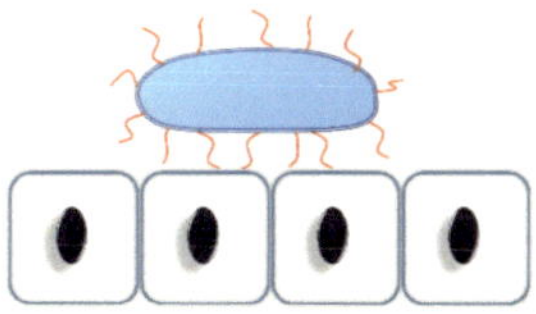	• SPAAN • FungalRV • MAAP
Antigenicity	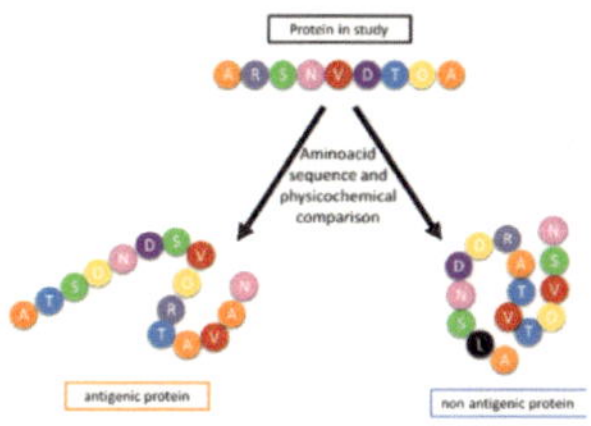	• VaxiJen • Protegen • EpiToolKit • SVMTriP
Similarity	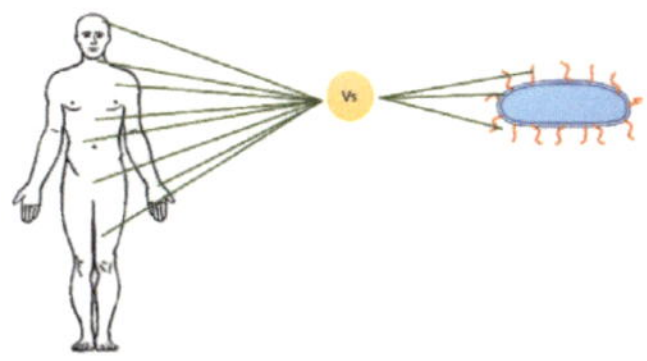	• BLAST
Transmembrane helix	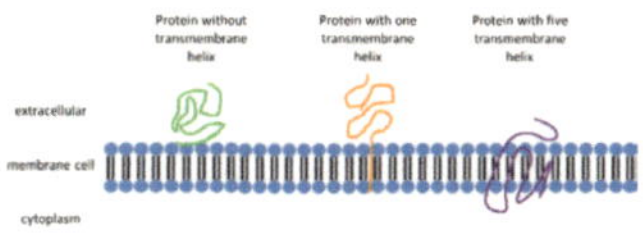	• TMHMM • TMpred • THGS • Sidekick • HMMTOP • SPLIT • DAS • Phobius • CCTOP • TMPad

Table 1. Main characteristics considered for vaccine candidate selection by reverse vaccinology.

3. Immunoinformatics

The immunological system can be classified as cellular or humoral and, depending on the disease, it can be induced the expected immune response. If a vaccine that induces a cellular response is needed, for example a tuberculosis vaccine [22] or a parasite vaccine against leishmaniasis [23], the software must search for antigens that can be recognized by the major histocompatibility complex (MHC) molecules present in T lymphocytes [4]. Software for this purpose include TEpredict, CTLPred, nHLAPred, ProPred-I, MAPPP, SVMHC, GPS-MBA, PREDIVAC, NetMHC, NetCTL, MHC2 Pred, IEDB, BIMAS, SVMHC, POPI, Epitopemap, iVAX, FRED2, Rankpep, BIMAS, PickPocket, KISS, and MHC2MIL. At their Websites, there are several options for search for MHC molecules as follows: for a specific species; type I or II, or even the allele(s) that will be employed for the prediction. The latter use different algorithms and some of these analyze the genome of the organism-under-study in order to identify new, probable MHC molecules.

On the other hand, if a humoral response is required, the software needs to identify antigens for B cells, for example, in the case of influenza virus or HIV [24, 25]. There is software that specifically searches for sequential epitopes for B cells, including BCPREDS, BepiPred, BEpro or PEPITO, ABCpred, Bcepred, IgPred, and BCEP. In addition, there are also Websites that, utilizing the 3D structure of a protein, can predict conformational epitopes for B cells, including the CEP, SEPPA, and DiscoTope Websites.

These software packages are based on computer training with the epitopes and nonepitopes previously identified, in order to provide values for new proteins and to predict whether or not it is an epitope. There are different techniques for this machine learning: position-specific scoring matrices (PSSMs), support vector machines (SVMs), hidden Markov models (HMMs), or artificial neural networks (ANNs). Each technique possesses different advantages and accuracy levels [26].

To achieve an analysis, the "immunome" of an organism is required; this includes all of the genes and proteins of cells that take part in its immune response. The study of all of the reactions that take part in the immune response is known as "immunomics" and it is specific for each organism; therefore, it is important to perform the study with information of the recipient organism. There have been many advances in the knowledge of immunomics using molecular biology and other throughput techniques, in order to understand the mechanisms of the immune system [27].

When immunomics and bioinformatics merged, a new science-denominated immunoinformatics was created, with the purpose of analyzing all of the information of an organism's immunomics and of making predictions of immune responses against specific molecules [28]. Websites already exist that present databases with antigens, with their epitopes identified in several organisms, and other immunological information, for example, IEDB, SIFPEITHI, IMGT, MHCBN, AntiJen, Dana-Farber Repository, and AgAbDb.

Once an antigen with the expected response has been identified, immunoinformatics can predict whether a region of an antigen, which usually is a protein, can generate a best stimulus by itself. If a protein has one epitope, this can be employed in a subunit vaccine and can be combined with other epitopes of different organisms in order to generate a polyvalent vaccine, reducing the cost of the formulation. The epitopes can be synthesized artificially or obtained with molecular biology tools. This renders a vaccine safer, not only in its formulation but also in its production process, because there is no risk of the presence of infectious organisms [29].

With the purpose of determining epitopes, the proteins are analyzed to identify hydrophilic regions. The tertiary structure of a protein is based on the interactions between the amino acids and the medium, that is, the region with hydrophilic amino acids is exposed to the exterior. In the opposite case, the hydrophobic amino acids are located in the center of the structure. If this protein interacts with immune cells, it is more probable that contact will be generated with the hydrophilic region, a place localized in the epitope [28].

An additional step can be added, that is the prediction of the stability of peptide binding to MHC, because some epitopes can be attached with greater force and affinity, making activation of the immune system more probable. For this purpose, software has been created such as NetMHCStab, which utilizes artificial networks for the analysis [30].

In the case of cancer vaccines, antigens present in B cell have been developed that can help in the cancer cell elimination process. Additionally, antibodies against regulatory T-cells have been found with aid in the regression process of the tumor [9, 31]. The latter opens the way in the search for epitopes that could be used in vaccines, allowing better and faster elimination of the disease. For an allergy vaccine, other predictors, such as Allermatch and AlgPred, can be employed with the purpose of identifying proteins with potential allergenicity.

Other software developers have addressed the analysis of the complete immune response against specific antigens, such as C-ImmSim. In this case, the software uses different algorithms for each step; at the end, a series of graphic representations of each cell type can supply an idea of whether the response is sufficient to protect against a disease [32]. However, the general panorama is limited because this analysis implies the interaction of many cells and molecules and, in many cases, we do not yet know how these can interact with each other in a specific disease.

4. Structural vaccinology

Structural vaccinology focuses on the conformational features of macromolecules, mainly proteins that make them good candidate antigens. This approach to vaccine design has been used mainly to select or design peptide-based vaccines or cross-reactive antigens with the capability of generating immunity against different antigenically divergent pathogens. The initial stage in bioinformatics analyses involves linear epitope prediction, taking hydrophilicity as the major characteristic for locating epitopes. However, considering these predictions as the sole factor in determining the potential of a sequence to be immunogenic is risky. For example, the predicted epitopes could be sterically hindered by nearby amino acids, or if a peptide vaccine is being developed, the resulting peptide could adopt a conformation that differs from the peptide within the context of a whole protein, resulting in different conformational epitopes. In fact, available structures from nonoclonal antibodies (Mab) complexed to proteins have demonstrated that, in the majority of cases, Mab recognize conformational rather than linear epitopes [33].

Many epitope-based vaccines attempt to elicit an antibody-mediated immune response that could neutralize the activity of toxins or pathogen receptors. Currently, there are many bioinformatics programs that predict protein epitopes. However, the majority of these programs rely only on the hydrophobicity or the hydrophilicity of amino acids. The main drawbacks in this are that many predicted epitopes are buried within the protein; thus, they would not be detected by the antibodies. In addition, the predicted epitopes are linear, leaving out conformational epitopes. In these cases, structural information can be helpful for selecting the epitopes that are exposed to the solvent and that are proximal to functional sites of the target protein, such as catalytic pockets or receptor binding pockets, or for detecting conformational epitopes on the surface of the target protein. Structural information is utilized to map antigenic epitopes to detect conformational features that could affect immunogenicity, such as the structural stability of proteins or the solvent exposure of candidate peptides, and to select antigenic regions shared by proteins of different pathogens that otherwise (i.e., by multiple alignments or epitope mapping) could not be evident. The approach that has been employed to develop vaccines is to perform several bioinformatics analyses at both at the sequence and structure level. For example, Cornick et al. [34] developed universal vaccine candidates against serotype 1 *Streptococcus pneumoniae* considering epitope prediction and structure modeling.

Protein flexibility can lead to vaccine failure due to high conformational variations that can avoid recognition by cell receptors or antibodies; for example, the failure of vaccines aimed at the HIV has been attributed to high flexibility of the globular head of gp120 [33, 35]. This is a concern, especially with peptides, which are usually more flexible and disordered than when they are found in a complete protein context. Bioinformatics predictions of flexibility can be attained from amino acid sequences (through structural alphabets) or from a 3D structure. High-performance bioinformatics tools such as molecular dynamics (MD) simulations can be employed to predict the stability of proteins or peptides [36]. This tool can be used to select the appropriate size of a peptide in order to render its stability and to introduce stabilizing mutations or chemical modifications that minimize flexibility, hence yielding better vaccine candidates than simple peptides.

Molecular docking is another bioinformatics tool that can be utilized in the selection and design of target antigens. It consists of complexing two molecules (protein-protein or protein-ligand) with best shape complementarity and minimal binding energy. In the field of structural vaccinology, molecular docking can be employed to predict the binding of epitopes to antibodies or to MHC receptors. Candidate antigens can be evaluated through the binding energy of the complex, and even mutations can be introduced to improve binding, but maintaining the specificity of the immune response [37].

Alam et al. [38], in a preliminary report, designed peptides as vaccine candidates against the Zika virus. They predicted MHC-I restricted epitopes, and then performed docking of these peptides with human leukocyte antigen (HLA) receptors to confirm their predictions. Toxicity analyses included allergenicity prediction. Another study proposed a multivalent vaccine with fused peptides against *Staphylococcus aureus*. Again, epitope prediction was followed by peptide structure prediction, docking with TLR2, molecular dynamics simulations to assess the stability of the complexes, and finally, allergenicity prediction [39].

Care should be taken while designing peptide-based vaccines because the resulting peptide could be toxic or allergenic. Several bioinformatics studies perform toxicity or allergenicity prediction on peptide candidates to rule out adverse effects in the resulting candidate vaccine [38, 39].

Bioinformatics analyses have been performed to improve the functionality of antibodies. One study modified the Fc portion of antibodies to increase binding of proteins to the antibodies' Fc. This approach is relevant to improve the functionality of designed antibodies, to study immune response evasion by some pathogens, and in biotechnology to purify antibodies or proteins [37].

One premise of bioinformatics is to detect epitopes that can be recognized by antibodies, but modeling antibody-antigen complexes has been difficult because of the mobility of protein loops in the Fab region of antibodies [40]. One way to avoid this drawback is the strategy presented by Koivuniemi et al., which involved homology modeling to deduce the structure of the antigen and the antibody, docking, and molecular dynamics simulations [41] (**Figure 1**).

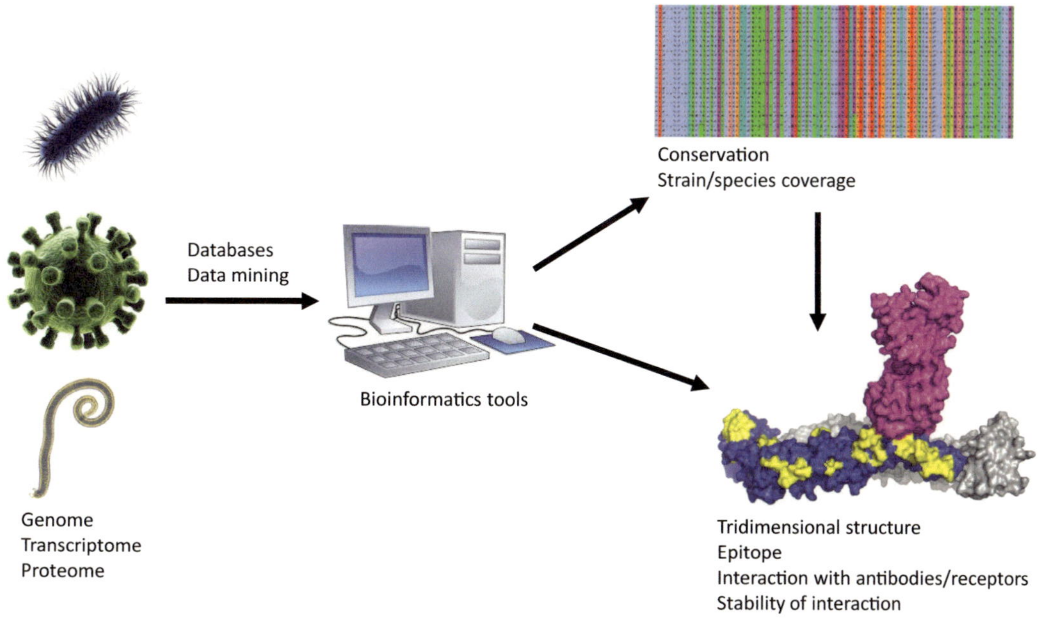

Figure 1. Path to antigen selection and validation. Databanks are created with experimental data from pathogens that can originate in the lab or be gathered through databases. Protein or nucleic acid sequences can be aligned to detect conservation and strain or species coverage. Three-dimensional (3D) structure information can be obtained from databases or inferred from bioinformatics analysis. Several predictions can be mapped into the structure, such as epitope prediction or amino acid conservation. Molecular docking tools can be used to establish interaction between two or more molecules (antibodies and cell receptors). Finally, the stability of these interactions can be assessed through energy calculations or molecular dynamics simulations.

5. Special cases: vaccines against infectious and noninfectious diseases

5.1. Vaccines against infectious diseases

5.1.1. Tuberculosis

Tuberculosis is an infectious disease caused by *Mycobacterium tuberculosis*, which is the most virulent and transmissible bacterium of the genus; however, it is a microorganism that is difficult to study because of its requirements and slow growth. The number of new cases worldwide rose to 10.4 million [42]; this high incidence rate is based on several factors, and one of the most important factors is the ineffectiveness of the vaccine used at present: the BCG. Thus, why many working groups are investigating new vaccines that can improve the level of protection against this disease, and one of the tools utilized is reverse vaccinology [10].

One strategy applied for vaccine design is to identify the structures present only in *M. tuberculosis* and absent in *Mycobacterium bovis* BCG [43]. In addition, the vaccine candidates studied presented the characteristics described previously, such as nonhuman homology, adhesins [44], secreted or membrane structures [45, 46] with low transmembrane helix, and in addition, the proteins expressed in the latent or active state of the microorganism [47]. The immunity sought is a protective response that is cellular. Therefore, immunoinformatics is based on the study of T-cell epitopes [22, 48–50].

Several candidates and epitopes have been found with different software. Some of these have been expressed and proven *in vitro* and *in vivo*, demonstrating their immunogenicity and protective effect. Among these are highlighted the ESAT-6, PE and PPE protein family group [51], and the Ag85 protein family, which obtained better immune response than the BCG vaccine in an animal model [43].

5.1.2. Influenza

The design of influenza vaccines is challenging due to the influenza virus's antigenic plasticity. Influenza viruses evade the immune response through antigenic drift and antigenic shift [52], rendering a long-lasting immune response very difficult. Current influenza vaccines contain hemagglutinin (HA) and neuraminidase (NA) as main antigenic components, usually having one type-B strain, and one H1 and one H3 subtype strain [53, 54]. Predicting the composition of next-year's vaccines relies on epidemiological data, although evolutionary models can aid in predicting antigenic drift, improving vaccine design [55].

Influenza HA recognizes cell receptors and mediates membrane fusion between the virus and the target cell. The globular head of HA contains the receptor binding site and the majority of the antigenic sites; consequently, this region is also the most variable. The stem region contains the fusion peptide and, although it previously was not considered a target for vaccine development, the discovery of neutralizing antibodies aimed at this region revealed its potential in vaccine design [52, 56]. Several conserved regions have been described in the stem region of HA [57], which make a universal vaccine a possibility. It has been found that neutralizing antibodies can bind to intact trimers, confirming the possibility of a universal vaccine aimed at the HA stem. In fact, engineered HA stem antigens have been shown to elicit immune responses against heterosubtypic challenge models and serve as a proof-of-concept that these vaccines work [58].

Given the high cooperation, hence availability, of influenza viral protein sequences, there are open databases such as OpenFluDB [59] or the Influenza Research Database [60] that help in the designing of influenza vaccines. EpiCombFlu is a database that aids in defining conserved epitopes across influenza strains that can be combined to maximize strain coverage. Analysis of these sequences has led to the identification of conserved motifs among influenza strains that can be targets in vaccine or inhibitor design [61].

5.1.3. Chikungunya fever

For CHIKungunya Virus (CHIKV), there are some vaccine candidates in clinical trials, but there is no licensed vaccine to date. Efforts include the development of vaccines of inactivated virus, live attenuated virus (LAV), and virus-like particles (VLPs). In preclinical studies, LAV and VLP vaccines have been promising, but during clinical trials, they have shown inadequate immunogenicity and residual virulence, for example, the risk of production of chronic rheumatism seen for LAV [62]. However, vaccines should be able to induce high levels of neutralizing antibodies, ideally with only one dose, LAV remain good candidates for which attenuation strategies are of central importance.

Because the CHIKV E2 glycoprotein is thought to interact with cellular receptors and has demonstrated to elicit neutralizing antibodies, generating protection against lethal challenge in mice [63], it has been extensively studied. Kam et al. [64] mapped its epitope-containing sequences using experimentally infected macaque antibodies. Their results revealed that one of four recognized regions mapped onto the surface of E2, that the majority of the epitopes clustered in the middle of the protein, and that antibody recognition of E2 changes throughout the disease course in experimentally infected macaques may be due to the spatial positions of the B-cell epitopes on the native form of the E1/E2 glycoprotein complex. As part of the study, these authors included computational modeling utilizing the structural data of the E2 retrieved from PDB and visualizing the results using UCSF CHIMERA software.

In the design of an LAV for CHIKV, Gardner et al. [65] considered three known facts: that the substitution for positively charged residues in E2 that confer enhanced, Heparan sulfate (HS)-dependent infectivity *in vitro* is a common phenomenon among cell culture-passaged strains of some CHIKV-related viruses; that these mutations can be selected from within only a few serial passages *in vitro*, and that viruses whose *in vitro* infectivity is enhanced by artificial HS attachment/entry are typically attenuated/avirulent *in vivo*. In the case of CHIKV, an LAV candidate, attenuated by serial passages in MRC-5 fibroblasts, the authors predicted an amino acid substitution at E2 position 82, which was highly dependent upon ionic interaction with HS for infectivity. Afterward, this mutation demonstrated the attenuation two strains of CHIKV *in vivo*. Based on this fact [59], E2 mutations were selected that confer HS dependence on infectivity by serial passage of wild-type CHIKV-LR on different cell types *in vitro*. Then they introduced these mutations individually into CHIKV and identified a panel of E2 mutations that confer reduced virulence in a murine model. In this work, computational modeling played an important role because it helped to explain the effect of the single amino acid mutations on altering the electrostatic profile of the E2 glycoprotein and increasing net positive charge in two exposed regions.

5.1.4. Zika virus disease

Zika virus, a positive single-stranded RNA virus transmitted by mosquito bites, is currently spreading worldwide and there is no available commercial vaccine. Several candidates are undergoing preclinical and clinical studies, and some platforms being investigated include inactivated, subunit/peptide, DNA-based, live-attenuated, and vectored vaccines. For a vaccine against this pathogen, multiple bioinformatics strategies are being exploited as an essential tool; the majority of studies involve *in silico* predictions to find the best epitopes. Dikhit et al. [66] found nine promiscuous highly conserved class I restricted epitopes among capsid 1, the envelope, and NS2A, NS4B, and NS5 viral proteins. Then, the tertiary structure of the selected epitopes was modeled using PEPstr and finally there was docking to HLA calculation with PatchDock.

Dar et al. [67] utilized ProPred1 to predict antigenic epitopes for HLA class I, as well as 48 antigenic epitopes for HLA class II employing ProPred immunoinformatics algorithms. These authors found 21% of MHC class I binding epitopes among NS5 viral proteins, followed by the envelope (17%). For MHC class II, NS5 contained 19% of predicted epitopes, and 17% were in the envelope, 17% in NS1, and 17% in NS2. Additionally, they obtained the antigenicity score for each predicted epitope using the VaxiJen 2.0 tool. Ashfaq and Ahmed are other researchers who used ProPred1 and ProPred, but focused in the envelope protein, finding two highly antigenic candidates among T-cell epitopes. They also performed a molecular docking to study the interactions of B-cell epitopes with HLA-B7 [68].

Another bioinformatics-based study is that of Mirza et al. [69], in which the authors predicted antigenic B-cell (IEDB) and CTL epitopes (NetCTL.1.2 server). They determined, by *in silico* studies, surface accessibility, surface flexibility, hydrophilicity, homology modeling (MODELLER ver. 9.12, CHARMM, WhatIF, PROCHECK, Verify 3D), and structure-based epitope prediction for E protein, NS3, and NS5. They performed molecular docking of the ZIKV-E protein with HLA-A0201, of the ZIKV-NS3 protein with HLA-B2705, and of the ZIKV-NS5 protein with HLA-C0801 (PatchDock rigid-body docking server, FireDock server). Finally, these authors investigated the stability of the docked peptide-MHC I protein complexes by performing Molecular Dynamics (MD) simulations (AMBER 12 simulation package) [69].

An important aspect in the design of a vaccine is the study of the virus's molecular biology, its proteome, and the genotypes. Sun et al. reported such data, to our knowledge for the first time, using new computational methods for annotation of mature peptide proteins, genotypes, and recombination events for all ZIKV genomes [70]. In an effort to aid in the development of vaccines and therapeutic drugs, an integrative multi-omics platform, ZikaVR (http://bioinfo.imtech.res.in/manojk/zikavr/) was created by Gupta el at.. This platform contains genomic, proteomic, and therapeutic information about the Zika virus [71].

5.2. Vaccines against noninfectious diseases

5.2.1. Vaccines to treat addictions

In the search for a vaccine to fight drug abuse, cocaine, nicotine, and methamphetamines are some of the main targets; however, to date there are, to our knowledge, no US: Federal Drug Administration (FDA)-approved vaccines. The development of such products has been hindered by the need of a carrier protein and an adjuvant to combine with haptens of the drugs to elicit the necessary antibody levels expected to interfere with the transport of the drug to the Central Nervous System (CNS), thus with the expected effect [72].

Kimishima et al. have explored tetanus toxoid (TT), the bacterial flagellin FliC, alum, and CpG (cytosine-phosphate-guanine oligodeoxynucleotide) in the development of an anticocaine vaccine. TT is used as a carrier; FliC acts as a carrier protein, and additionally it has been demonstrated that it stimulates toll-like receptor 5 (TLR5), therefore inducing myeloid differentiation factor 88 (MyD88), which renders a TH2 response to predominant production of IgG1 and no cytotoxic T lymphocytes (CTL). CpG (a B-class OligoDeoxyNucleotide [ODN]) motifs can be used as activators of TLR9 to promote a TH1-type immune response, stimulating B-cell immune responses to generate IgG2a and CTL [73].

Lockner et al., in a first attempt, conjugated GNE (a cocaine hapten) with a recombinant FliC, utilized *in silico* modeling and computational analysis of the recombinant protein to ensure its structural integrity and conservation of the binding to TLR5; by Modeler, they studied the homology of the recombinant flagellin, as well as the number of lysines per domain and relative solvent accessibility with and without GNE cocaine haptens present. Their computational results agreed with those used for experimentation since then in a TLR5 reporter assay: the modified flagellin protein still activated TLR5 when the hapten density was <10 GNE per FliC. Finally, the authors showed that cocaine-flagellin conjugates induced, in a dose-dependent model, the production of anticocaine antibodies in mice, improving the response with the adjuvant alum [73, 74].

On the other hand, as they observed in prior experiments in which they conjugated GNE (a cocaine hapten) with FliC, TLR5 activation was attenuated at higher hapten densities (i.e., above $\sim$10 GNE per flagellin). Consequently, they induced a mutation in the flagellin gene (*mFliC*), which could protect the TLR5 binding interface against covalent modification with the bulky GNE hapten, thus potentially preserving the ability of the modified flagellin to activate TLR5 independently of hapten densities. *mFliC* consisted of a mutation of the 10 lysine residues within the D0 and D1 domains of wild-type *FliC* (as well as one additional lysine residue previously introduced through cloning) to arginine residues [73]. Again, bioinformatics was necessary to assess the secondary structure and MHC-II binding predictions for FliC and mFliC, employing the PSIPRED (http://bioinf.cs.ucl.ac.uk/psipred/) method and the external software from IEDB (http://www.immuno-epitope.org/), respectively [74].

The computational results for MHC-II binding and hapten presentation revealed that the FliC conjugate was better than mFliC; these results indirectly correlated with those conducted by enzyme-linked immunosorbent assays (ELISA) and radioimmunoassays (RIA). However, because FliC and mFliC exhibited poor efficacy as carrier proteins when comparing two formulations, GNE-FliC + CpG and GNE-TT + CpG, through a hyperlocomotion test and analysis of cocaine in blood, where GNE-TT + CpG had best efficacy, the authors proposed the investigation of monomers of FliC instead of the polymeric form utilized [74].

5.2.1.1. Allergies

Allergies comprise another area where vaccine (specific immunotherapy (SIT)) investigation is conferred due to the association of allergy with asthma and anaphylaxis. Some common allergies are caused by cat, peanut, and cockroach allergens, with the specific immunotherapy (SIT) effective, but sometimes associated with IgE-dependent adverse events. In allergies, computational approaches have been applied to find T-cell epitopes to target allergen-specific T cells, thus improving the safety of the immunotherapy.

In 2011, Worm et al. performed a clinical study administering the ToleroMune cat vaccine (short synthetic peptide sequences from the major cat allergen Fel d 1) to 66 subjects with cat allergy. The authors identified each peptide-MHC interaction by using physical binding assays and analyzed these *in silico* with the immune epitope database (www.immuneepitope.org/); *in vitro*, the individual peptides and the vaccine were at least 1000-fold less able to induce basophil histamine release associated with adverse effects than the native allergen. The vaccine administered intradermally (i.d.) or subcutaneously (s.c.) showed no serious adverse events (SAEs) during the study and no subject withdrew from the latter due to an adverse event. Thus, the vaccine was safe and well tolerated [75].

Another example of research to improve safety comprises the work of Pascal et al. for the treatment of peanut allergy, which presents symptoms ranging from mild oropharyngeal pruritus to life-threatening anaphylaxis, considerably compromising the patient's quality of life. Ara h 1, Ara h 2, and Ara h 3 include the three major peanut allergens, although IgE antibodies to Ara h 2 correlate most closely with clinical reactivity, and *in vitro* Ara h 2 and its homologue, Ara h 6, are more potent inducers of basophil degranulation than Ara h 1 and Ara h 3. Because conventional s.c. immunotherapy with crude peanut extract entertains a high risk of anaphylaxis and since peptides have been successful in the desensitization of patients to cat-allergy and bee venom-allergy, an alternative is the use of peptide fragments that retain immunogenicity, but that are of insufficient length to cross-link allergen-specific IgE on mast cells and basophils. In addition to proliferation assays utilizing peripheral blood mononuclear cells (PBMCs) from peanut-allergic children and Ara h 2 peptides, Pascal and colleagues predicted, to our knowledge for the first-time, epitopes in a food-allergy through the artificial neural network-based alignment (NN-align) method NetMHCIIpan-2.0. Their objective was to analyze additional theoretical peptides that are not included in the proliferation assays, finding that both strategies, *in vitro* and *in silico,* rendered consistent results; therefore, they were able to select peptide candidates for the development of a peanut allergy vaccine [76].

Regarding allergy to cockroaches, there are some research studies that have followed the *in silico* prediction of B-cell, T-cell, and IgE-binding epitopes in a first stage to propose a vaccine formulation. Chen et al., Yang et al., and Tong et al. are members of a workgroup that studied this allergy by means of *in vitro* and *in silico* approaches. The allergens analyzed were Per a 6 and Bla g (found in *Periplaneta americana* and *Blattella germanica*, respectively) [77–79].

Chen et al. employed three immunoinformatics tools: the Protean™ system (DNAStar, Inc., Madison, WI, USA); the bioinformatics predicted antigenic peptides (BPAP) system (http://imed.med.ucm.es/Tools/antigenic.pl), and the BepiPred 1.0 server (http://www.cbs.dtu.dk/services/BepiPred/), which utilizes four properties, including hydrophilicity, flexibility, accessibility, and antigenicity as parameters for the prediction of B-cell epitopes. After a consensus of the three bioinformatics tools, these authors selected the final potential epitope regions (regions whose consensus epitope result was 67 or 100%) to develop a vaccine. Additionally, through the NN-align method NetMHCIIpan-2.0 (http://www.cbs.dtu.dk/services/NetMHCIIpan/) for HLA-DR alleles and NetMHCII-2.2 (http://www.cbs.dtu.dk/services/NetMHCII/) for HLA-DQ alleles, they found strong and weak binders [77]. In 2016, Yang et al. and Tong et al. predicted, using the same strategy, B- and T-cell peptides belonging to Per a 9 and Per a 10 (two major allergens as assessed by enzyme-linked immunosorbent assays (ELISA) but, in order to obtain substantial quantities of these allergens for use in functional studies, they cloned and expressed them in an *Escherichia coli* system [78, 79]

5.2.1.2. Cancer

Since T cells educated in the thymus do not recognize mutated antigens expressed in cancer cells, there is no negative selection, and these neoantigens are ideal targets for therapeutic vaccination; furthermore, they are not present in healthy tissue. On the other hand, advances in next-generation sequencing (NGS) permit the sequencing of genomes, exomes, or transcriptomes within hours. Therefore, they investigated the mutanome (the tens-to-hundreds of somatic nonsynonymous mutations) in order to select the specific targets for the recognition by cytotoxic and helper T cells with antitumor activity. The complexity of some experimental tools such as mass spectrometry hampers its usefulness in the selection of targets in a clinical setting where personalized therapy is needed. In this context, because it is not possible to analyze all of the mutations, bioinformatics addresses this problem and has become important in the selection of targets and in their prioritization [80].

An example of the success of *in silico* predicted mutations is the study of Castle et al., where the authors, applying thresholds for MHC class II binding prediction and mRNA expression levels, without further validation by immunogenicity testing, were able to enrich immunogenic MHC class II-restricted epitopes. They obtained efficient and sustained control of advanced tumors in mice [81].

Although there are successful *in vitro* and preclinical studies that initiated by utilizing computational approaches, the majority of algorithms predict the affinity of peptide binding to MHC molecules, which may not correlate well with their immunogenicity or may not predict peptides that are not generated and presented. Moreover, some immunogenic ligands may escape detection. Additionally, in general *in silico* prediction of ligands for MHC II is less accurate than for MHC molecules. Because the immunogenicity of predicted peptides has been reported to correlate better with peptide-MHC complex stability, the use has been proposed of biochemical methods to reduce the number of *in silico* predicted MHC ligands and to generate data that helps in the training of prediction algorithms to validate peptide binding predictions. Some biochemical methods include peptide rebinding (referred to as iTopia), peptide-rescuing, and refolding for MHC I peptide binding validation, and peptide-driven refolding for MHC II [82].

Another approach to circumvent the limitations of the binding prediction for MHC molecules is molecular docking, a structure-based method that has been tested on both peptide-MHC class I and II complexes. This method can be applied to previously predicted peptides and is expected to improve prediction accuracy in order to identify the best MHC class I and II binders. Following this strategy, in a research for vaccine candidates against breast cancer, predicted discontinuous B-cell epitope peptides using PEPOP for the first time, then the 3D structure of epitope-based peptides by PEP-FOLD server, and their theoretical physicochemical properties utilizing the Prot Param algorithm, and finally, with.pdb files of two class I and seven class II MHC-peptide complexes from the protein data bank, perform molecular docking through the genetic optimization for ligand docking (GOLD) 5.4. After virtual screening, they confirmed a predicted peptide agreement between their docked results and previous experimental results (i.e., the immunogenicity of this peptide was confirmed *in vivo* studies), thus proposing molecular docking as an additional technique to improve the selection of peptide candidates for cancer vaccines [83].

Acknowledgements

The authors are grateful for the support of this work from Instituto Politécnico Nacional (IPN) Grants SIP-IPN 20171932, 20172085, 20171766, and 20171992. RMR-A and GA-O thank EDD-IPN; JAC-V and AJ-A thank EDI-IPN. All authors are grateful to COFAA-IPN. Authors thank Margaret Brunner for English editing.

Author details

Ribas-Aparicio Rosa María[1]*, Castelán-Vega Juan Arturo[1], Jiménez-Alberto Alicia[1], Monterrubio-López Gloria Paulina[1] and Aparicio-Ozores Gerardo[2]

*Address all correspondence to: rribas233@yahoo.com

1 Laboratory of Production and Biological Control, Department of Microbiology, National School of Biological Sciences, National Polytechnic Institute, Mexico City, Mexico

2 Laboratory of Medical Bacteriology, Department of Microbiology, National School of Biological Sciences, National Polytechnic Institute, Mexico City, Mexico

References

[1] Plotkin ST, Plotkin SA. A short history of vaccination. In: Plotkin SA, Orenstein WA, Offit PA, editors. Vaccines. 6th ed. Philadelphia, PA, USA: Elsevier/Saunders; 2013. pp. 1-13

[2] Bulletin of the World Health Organization (WHO). Available from: http://www.who.int/bulletin/volumes/86/2/07-040089/en/

[3] Rappuoli R. Reverse vaccinology. Current Opinion in Microbiology. 2000;**3**(5):445-450

[4] He Y, Rappuoli R, De Groot AS, Chen RT. Emerging vaccine informatics. Journal of Biomedicine and Biotechnology. 2010;**2010**:218590. DOI: 10.1155/2010/218590

[5] Welly BT, Miller MR, Stott JL, Blanchard MT, Islas-Trejo AD, O'Rourke SM, Young AE, Medrano JF, Van Eenennaam AL. Genome report: Identification and validation of antigenic proteins from *Pajaroellobacter abortibovis* using *de novo* genome sequence assembly and reverse vaccinology. G3 (Bethesda). 2017;**7**(2):321-331. DOI: 10.1534/g3.116.036673

[6] Plotkin S. History of vaccination. Proceedings of the National Academy of Sciences of the United States. 2014;**111**(34):12283-12287. DOI: 10.1073/pnas.1400472111

[7] Seib KL, Zhao X, Rappuoli R. Developing vaccines in the era of genomics: A decade of reverse vaccinology. Clinical Microbiology and Infection. 2012;**18**(Suppl 5):109-116. DOI: 10.1111/j.1469-0691.2012.03939.x

[8] Vivona S, Bernante F, Filippini F. NERVE: New enhanced reverse vaccinology environment. BMC Biotechnology. 2006;**6**:35

[9] Delany I, Rappuoli R, De Gregorio E. Vaccines for the 21st century. EMBO Molecular Medicine. 2014;**6**(6):708-720. DOI: 10.1002/emmm.201403876

[10] Monterrubio-López GP, González-Y-Merchand JA, Ribas-Aparicio RM. Identification of novel potential vaccine candidates against tuberculosis Based on reverse vaccinology. BioMed Research International. 2015;**2015**:483150. DOI: 10.1155/2015/483150

[11] Jaiswal V, Chanumolu SK, Gupta A, Chauhan RS, Rout C. Jenner-predict server: Prediction of protein vaccine candidates (PVCs) in bacteria based on host-pathogen interactions. BMC Bioinformatics. 2013;**14**:211. DOI: 10.1186/1471-2105-14-211

[12] Pizza M, Scarlato V, Masignani V, Giuliani MM, Aricò B, Comanducci M, Jennings GT, Baldi L, Bartolini E, Capecchi B, Galeotti CL, Luzzi E, Manetti R, Marchetti E, Mora M, Nuti S, Ratti G, Santini L, Savino S, Scarselli M, Storni E, Zuo P, Broeker M, Hundt E, Knapp B, Blair E, Mason T, Tettelin H, Hood DW, Jeffries AC, Saunders NJ, Granoff DM, Venter JC, Moxon ER, Grandi G, Rappuoli R. Identification of vaccine candidates against serogroup B meningococcus by whole-genome sequencing. Science. 2000;**287**(5459):1816-1820

[13] Lew-Tabor AE, Rodríguez-Valle M. A review of reverse vaccinology approaches for the development of vaccines against ticks and tick borne diseases. Ticks and Tick-borne Diseases. 2016;**7**(4):573-585. DOI: 10.1016/j.ttbdis.2015.12.012

[14] Goodswen SJ, Kennedy PJ, Ellis JT. A guide to *in silico* vaccine discovery for eukaryotic pathogens. Briefings in Bioinformatics. 2013;**14**(6):753-774. DOI: 10.1093/bib/bbs066

[15] Chaudhuri R, Kulshreshtha D, Raghunandanan MV, Ramachandran S. Integrative immunoinformatics for Mycobacterial diseases in R platform. Systems and Synthetic Biology. 2014;**8**(1):27-39. DOI: 10.1007/s11693-014-9135-9

[16] Chaudhuri R, Ramachandran S. Prediction of virulence factors using bioinformatics approaches. Methods in Molecular Biology. 2014;**1184**:389-400. DOI: 10.1007/978-1-4939-1115-8_22

[17] Sachdeva G, Kumar K, Jain P, Ramachandran S. SPAAN: A software program for prediction of adhesins and adhesin-like proteins using neural networks. Bioinformatics. 2005;**21**(4):483-491

[18] Doytchinova IA, Flower DR. VaxiJen: A server for prediction of protective antigens, tumour antigens and subunit vaccines. BMC Bioinformatics. 2007;**8**:4

[19] Argondizzo AP, da Mota FF, Pestana CP, Reis JN, de Miranda AB, Galler R, Medeiros MA. Identification of proteins in *Streptococcus pneumoniae* by reverse vaccinology and genetic diversity of these proteins in clinical isolates. Applied Biochemistry and Biotechnology. 2015;**175**(4):2124-2165. DOI: 10.1007/s12010-014-1375-3

[20] Altindis E, Cozzi R, Di Palo B, Necchi F, Mishra RP, Fontana MR, Soriani M, Bagnoli F, Maione D, Grandi G, Liberatori S. Protectome analysis: A new selective bioinformatics tool for bacterial vaccine candidate discovery. Molecular & Cellular Proteomics. 2015;**14**(2):418-429. DOI: 10.1074/mcp.M114.039362

[21] Meunier M, Guyard-Nicodème M, Hirchaud E, Parra A, Chemaly M, Dory D. Identification of novel vaccine candidates against *Campylobacter* through reverse vaccinology. Journal of Immunology Research. 2016;**2016**:5715790. DOI: 10.1155/2016/5715790

[22] Pandey K, Sharma M, Saarav I, Singh S, Dutta P, Bhardwaj A, Sharma S. Analysis of the DosR regulon genes to select cytotoxic T lymphocyte epitope specific vaccine candidates using a reverse vaccinology approach. International Journal of Mycobacteriology. 2016;**5**(1):34-43. DOI: 10.1016/j.ijmyco.2015.10.005

[23] Seyed N, Taheri T, Rafati S. Post-genomics and vaccine improvement for *Leishmania*. Frontiers in Microbiology. 2016;**7**:467. DOI: 10.3389/fmicb.2016.00467

[24] Rappuoli R, Bottomley MJ, D'Oro U, Finco O, De Gregorio E. Reverse vaccinology 2.0: Human immunology instructs vaccine antigen design. Journal of Experimental Medicine. 2016;**213**(4):469-481. DOI: 10.1084/jem.20151960

[25] Van Regenmortel MH. An outdated notion of antibody specificity is one of the major detrimental assumptions of the structure-based reverse vaccinology paradigm, which prevented it from helping to develop an effective HIV-1 vaccine. Frontiers in Immunology. 2014;**5**:593. DOI: 10.3389/fimmu.2014.00593

[26] Backert L, Kohlbacher O. Immunoinformatics and epitope prediction in the age of genomic medicine. Genome Medicine. 2015;**7**:119. DOI: 10.1186/s13073-015-0245-0

[27] Tomar N, De RK. Immunoinformatics: A brief review. Methods in Molecular Biology. 2014;**1184**:23-55. DOI: 10.1007/978-1-4939-1115-8_3

[28] Flower DR. Vaccines: Data driven prediction of binders, epitope and immunogenicity. In: Bioinformatics for Vaccinology. United Kingdom: Wiley-Blackwell; 2008. pp. 167-215

[29] Delany I, Rappuoli R, Seib KL. Vaccines, reverse vaccinology, and bacterial pathogenesis. Cold Spring Harbor Perspectives in Medicine. 2013;**3**(5):a012476. DOI: 10.1101/cshperspect.a012476

[30] Jørgensen KW, Rasmussen M, Buus S, Nielsen M. NetMHCstab- predicting stability of peptide-MHC-I complexes; impacts for cytotoxic T lymphocyte epitope discovery. Immunology. 2014;**141**(1):18-26. DOI: 10.1111/imm.12160

[31] Rappuoli R, Pizza M, Del Giudice G, De Gregorio E. Vaccines, new opportunities for a new society. Proceedings of the National Academy of Sciences of the United States. 2014;**111**(34):12288-12293. DOI: 10.1073/pnas.1402981111

[32] Rapin N, Lund O, Bernaschi M, Castiglione F. Computational immunology meets bioinformatics: The use of prediction tools for molecular binding in the simulation of the immune system. PLOS ONE. 2010;**5**(4):e9862. DOI: 10.1371/journal.pone.0009862

[33] Van Regenmortel MH. Structure-based reverse vaccinology failed in the case of HIV because it disregarded accepted immunological theory. International Journal of Molecular Sciences. 2016;**17**(9):1591

[34] Cornick JE, Tastan Bishop Ö, Yalcin F, Kiran AM, Kumwenda B, Chaguza C, Govindpershad S, Ousmane S, Senghore M, du Plessis M, Pluschke G, Ebruke C, McGee L, Sigaùque B, Collard JM, Bentley SD, Kadioglu A, Antonio M, von Gottberg A, French N, Klugman KP, Heyderman RS, Alderson M, Everett DB; PAGe Consortium. The global distribution and diversity of protein vaccine candidate antigens in the highly virulent *Streptococcus pneumoniae* serotype 1. Vaccine. 2017;**35**(6):972-980. DOI: 10.1016/j.vaccine.2016.12.037

[35] Korkut A, Hendrickson WA. Structural plasticity and conformational transitions of HIV envelope glycoprotein gp120. PLOS ONE. 2012;**7**(12):e52170. DOI: 10.1371/journal.pone.0052170

[36] Zhu Z, Zhang C, Song W. Rational derivation, extension, and cyclization of self-inhibitory peptides to target TGF-β/BMP signaling in ONFH. Amino Acids. 2017;**49**(2):283-290. DOI: 10.1007/s00726-016-2358-1

[37] Agostino M, Mancera RL, Ramsland PA, Fernández-Recio J. Optimization of protein-protein docking for predicting Fc-protein interactions. Journal of Molecular Recognition. 2016;**29**(11):555-568. DOI: 10.1002/jmr.2555

[38] Alam A, Ali S, Ahamad S, Malik MZ, Ishrat R. From ZikV genome to vaccine: *In silico* approach for the epitope-based peptide vaccine against Zika virus envelope glycoprotein. Immunology. 2016;**149**(4):386-399. DOI: 10.1111/imm.12656

[39] Hajighahramani N, Nezafat N, Eslami M, Negahdaripour M, Rahmatabadi SS, Ghasemi Y. Immunoinformatics analysis and *in silico* designing of a novel multi-epitope peptide vaccine against *Staphylococcus aureus*. Infection, Genetics and Evolution. 2016;**48**:83-94. DOI: 10.1016/j.meegid.2016.12.010

[40] Bohnuud T, Luo L, Wodak SJ, Bonvin AM, Weng Z, Vajda S, Schueler-Furman O, Kozakov D. A benchmark testing ground for integrating homology modeling and protein docking. Proteins. 2017;**85**(1):10-16. DOI: 10.1002/prot.25063

[41] Koivuniemi A, Takkinen K, Nevanen T. A computational approach for studying antibody-antigen interactions without prior structural information: The anti-testosterone binding antibody as a case study. Proteins. 2017;**85**(2):322-331. DOI: 10.1002/prot.25226

[42] World Health Organization. Global Tuberculosis Report; 2016

[43] Mollenkopf HJ, Grode L, Mattow J, Stein M, Mann P, Knapp B, Ulmer J, Kaufmann SH. Application of mycobacterial proteomics to vaccine design: Improved protection by *Mycobacterium bovis* BCG prime-Rv3407 DNA boost vaccination against tuberculosis. Infection and Immunity. 2004;**72**(11):6471-6479

[44] Kumar S, Puniya BL, Parween S, Nahar P, Ramachandran S. Identification of novel adhesins of *M. tuberculosis* H37Rv using integrated approach of multiple computational algorithms and experimental analysis. PLOS ONE. 2013;**8**(7):e69790. DOI: 10.1371/journal.pone.0069790

[45] Vizcaíno C, Restrepo-Montoya D, Rodríguez D, Niño LF, Ocampo M, Vanegas M, Reguero MT, Martínez NL, Patarroyo ME, Patarroyo MA. Computational prediction and experimental assessment of secreted/surface proteins from *Mycobacterium tuberculosis* H37Rv. PLOS Computational Biology. 2010;**6**(6):e1000824. DOI: 10.1371/journal.pcbi.1000824

[46] Song H, Sandie R, Wang Y, Andrade-Navarro MA, Niederweis M. Identification of outer membrane proteins of *Mycobacterium tuberculosis*. Tuberculosis (Edinburgh). 2008;**88**(6):526-544. DOI: 10.1016/j.tube.2008.02.004

[47] Nguyen Thi le T, Sarmiento ME, Calero R, Camacho F, Reyes F, Hossain MM, González GS, Norazmi MN, Acosta A. Immunoinformatics study on highly expressed *Mycobacterium tuberculosis* genes during infection. Tuberculosis (Edinburgh). 2014;**94**(5):475-481

[48] Sundaramurthi JC, Brindha S, Shobitha SR, Swathi A, Ramanandan P, Hanna LE. *In silico* identification of potential antigenic proteins and promiscuous CTL epitopes in *Mycobacterium tuberculosis*. Infection, Genetics and Evolution. 2012;**12**(6):1312-1318. DOI: 10.1016/j.meegid.2012.03.023

[49] Vani J, Shaila MS, Chandra NR, Nayak R. A combined immuno-informatics and structure-based modeling approach for prediction of T cell epitopes of secretory proteins of Mycobacterium tuberculosis. Microbes and Infection. 2006;**8**(3):738-746

[50] Tang ST, van Meijgaarden KE, Caccamo N, Guggino G, Klein MR, van Weeren P, Kazi F, Stryhn A, Zaigler A, Sahin U, Buus S, Dieli F, Lund O, Ottenhoff TH. Genome-based *in silico* identification of new *Mycobacterium tuberculosis* antigens activating polyfunctional CD8+ T cells in human tuberculosis. Journal of Immunology. 2011;**186**(2):1068-1080. DOI: 10.4049/jimmunol.1002212

[51] Pajón R, Yero D, Lage A, Llanes A, Borroto CJ. Computational identification of beta-barrel outer-membrane proteins in *Mycobacterium tuberculosis* predicted proteomes as putative vaccine candidates. Tuberculosis (Edinburgh). 2006;**86**(3-4):290-302

[52] Bouvier NM, Palese P. The biology of influenza viruses. Vaccine. 2008;**26**(Suppl 4):D49-D53

[53] Lambach P, Álvarez AM, Hirve S, Ortiz JR, Hombach J, Verweij M, Hendriks J, Palkonyay L, Pfleiderer M. Considerations of strategies to provide influenza vaccine year round. Vaccine. 2015;**33**(47):6493-6498. DOI: 10.1016/j.vaccine.2015.08.037

[54] Alan H, Ian B, Nancy C, Ruben OD, Siddhivinayak H, Daniel J, Jacqueline K, John M, Fernando M, Takato O, Tam JS, Anthony W, Richard W, Thedi Z, Wenqing Z. Improving the selection and development of influenza vaccine viruses—Report of a WHO informal consultation on improving influenza vaccine virus selection, Hong Kong SAR, China, 18-20 November 2015. Vaccine. 2017;**35**(8):1104-1109. DOI: 10.1016/j.vaccine.2017.01.018

[55] Xu H, Yang Y, Wang S, Zhu R, Qiu T, Qiu J, Zhang Q, Jin L, He Y, Tang K, Cao Z. Predicting the mutating distribution at antigenic sites of the influenza virus. Scientific Reports. 2016;**6**:20239. DOI: 10.1038/srep20239

[56] Neu KE, Henry Dunand CJ, Wilson PC. Heads, stalks and everything else: How can antibodies eradicate influenza as a human disease? Current Opinion in Immunology. 2016;**42**:48-55. DOI: 10.1016/j.coi.2016.05.012

[57] Harris AK, Meyerson JR, Matsuoka Y, Kuybeda O, Moran A, Bliss D, Das SR, Yewdell JW, Sapiro G, Subbarao K, Subramaniam S. Structure and accessibility of HA trimers on intact 2009 H1N1 pandemic influenza virus to stem region-specific neutralizing antibodies. Proceedings of the National Academy of Sciences of the United States. 2013;**110**(12):4592-4597. DOI: 10.1073/pnas.1214913110

[58] Impagliazzo A, Milder F, Kuipers H, Wagner MV, Zhu X, Hoffman RM, van Meersbergen R, Huizingh J, Wanningen P, Verspuij J, de Man M, Ding Z, Apetri A, Kükrer B, Sneekes-Vriese E, Tomkiewicz D, Laursen NS, Lee PS, Zakrzewska A, Dekking L, Tolboom J, Tettero L, van Meerten S, Yu W, Koudstaal W, Goudsmit J, Ward AB, Meijberg W, Wilson IA, Radošević K. A stable trimeric influenza hemagglutinin stem as a broadly protective immunogen. Science. 2015;**349**(6254):1301-1306. DOI: 10.1126/science.aac7263

[59] Liechti R, Gleizes A, Kuznetsov D, Bougueleret L, Le Mercier P, Bairoch A, Xenarios I. OpenFluDB, a database for human and animal influenza virus. Database (Oxford). 2010;**2010**:baq004. DOI: 10.1093/database/baq004

[60] Zhang Y, Aevermann BD, Anderson TK, Burke DF, Dauphin G, Gu Z, He S, Kumar S, Larsen CN, Lee AJ, Li X, Macken C, Mahaffey C, Pickett BE, Reardon B, Smith T, Stewart L, Suloway C, Sun G, Tong L, Vincent AL, Walters B, Zaremba S, Zhao H, Zhou L, Zmasek C, Klem EB, Scheuermann RH. Influenza research database: An integrated bioinformatics resource for influenza virus research. Nucleic Acids Research. 2017;**45**(D1):D466-D474. DOI: 10.1093/nar/gkw857

[61] ElHefnawi M, Alaidi O, Mohamed N, Kamar M, El-Azab I, Zada S, Siam R. Identification of novel conserved functional motifs across most Influenza A viral strains. Virology Journal. 2011;**8**:44. DOI: 10.1186/1743-422X-8-44

[62] Singh P, Chhabra M, Mittal V, Sharma P, Rizvi MA, Chauhan LS, Rai A. Current research and clinical trials for a vaccine against chikungunya virus. Vaccine: Development and Therapy. 2013;**3**:35-46. DOI: https://doi.org/10.2147/VDT.S25513

[63] van den Doel P, Volz A, Roose JM, Sewbalaksing VD, Pijlman GP, Middelkoop I, Duiverman V, Wetering E, Sutter G, Osterhaus ADME, Martina BEE. Recombinant modified vaccinia virus ankara expressing glycoprotein E2 of chikungunya virus protects AG129 mice against lethal challenge. PLOS Neglected Tropical Diseases. 2014;**8**(9):e3101. DOI: 10.1371/journal.pntd.0003101

[64] Kam Y-W, Lee WWL, Simarmata D, Le Grand R, Tolou H, Merits A, Roques P, Ng LFP. Unique epitopes recognized by antibodies induced in chikungunya virus-infected non-human primates: Implications for the study of immunopathology and vaccine development. PLOS ONE. 2014;**9**(4):e95647. DOI: 10.1371/journal.pone.0095647

[65] Gardner CL, Hritz J, Sun C, Vanlandingham DL, Song TY, Ghedin E, Higgs S, Klimstra WB, Ryman KD. Deliberate attenuation of chikungunya virus by adaptation to Heparan sulfate-dependent infectivity: A model for rational arboviral vaccine design. PLOS Neglected Tropical Diseases. 2014;**8**(2):e2719. DOI: 10.1371/journal.pntd.0002719

[66] Dikhit MR, Ansari MY, Vijaymahantesh, Kalyani, Mansuri R, Sahoo BR, Dehury B, Amit A, Topnof RK, Sahoo GC, Ali V, Bimal S, Das P. Computational prediction and analysis of potential antigenic CTL epitopes in Zika virus: A first step towards vaccine development. Infection, Genetics and Evolution. 2016;**45**:187-197. DOI: org/10.1016/j.meegid.2016.08.037 DOI: 10.1016/j.meegid.2016.08.037

[67] Dar H, Zaheer T, Rehman MT, Ali A, Javed A, Khan GA, Babar MM, Waheed Y. Prediction of promiscuous T-cell epitopes in the Zika virus polyprotein: An *in silico* approach. Asian Pacific Journal of Tropical Disease. 2016;**9**(9):844-850. DOI: org/10.1016/j.apjtm.2016.07.004

[68] Ashfaq UA, Ahmed B. *De novo* structural modeling and conserved epitopes prediction of Zika virus envelope protein for vaccine development. Viral Immunology. 2016;**29**(7):436-443. DOI: 10.1089/vim.2016.0033

[69] Mirza MU, Rafique S, Ali A, Munir M, Ikram N, Manan A, Salo-Ahen OMH, Idrees M. Zika virus: Immunoinformatics combined with molecular dynamics simulations to predict antigenic epitopes of Zika viral proteins. Scientific Reports. 2016;**6**:37313. DOI: 10.1038/srep37313

[70] Sun G, Larsen CN, Baumgarth N, Klem EB, Scheuermann RH. Comprehensive annotation of mature peptides and genotypes for Zika virus. PLOS ONE. 2017;**12**(1):e0170462. DOI: 10.1371/journal.pone.0170462

[71] Gupta AK, Kaur K, Rajput A, Dhanda SK, Sehgal M, Khan MdS, Monga I, Dar SA, Singh S, Nagpal G, Usmani SS, Thakur A, Kaur G, Sharma S, Bhardwaj A, Qureshi A, Raghava GPS, Kumar M. ZikaVR. An integrated Zika virus resource for genomics, proteomics, phylogenetic and therapeutic analysis. Scientific Reports. 2016;**6**:32713. DOI: 10.1038/srep32713

[72] National Institute on Drug Abuse. NIH, USA. Available from: https://www.drugabuse.gov/

[73] Kimishima A, Wenthur CJ, Eubanks LM, Sato S, Janda KD. Cocaine vaccine development: Evaluation of carrier and adjuvant combinations that activate multiple Toll-Like receptors. Molecular Pharmaceutics. 2016;**13**:3884-3890

[74] Lockner JW, Eubanks LM, Choi JL, Lively JM, Schlosburg JE, Collins KC, Globisch D, Rosenfeld-Gunn RJ, Wilson IA, Janda KD. Flagellin as carrier and adjuvant in cocaine vaccine development. Molecular Pharmaceutics. 2015;**12**:653-662. DOI: 10.1021/mp500520r

[75] Worm M, Lee H-H, Kleine-Tebbe J, Hafner RP, Laidler P, Healey D, Buhot C, Verhoef A, Maillere B, Kay AB, Larché M. Development and preliminary clinical evaluation of a peptide immunotherapy vaccine for cat allergy. The Journal of Allergy and Clinical Immunology. 2011;**127**:89-97. DOI: 10.1016/j.jaci.2010.11.029

[76] Pascal M, Konstantinou GN, Masilamani M, Lieberman J, Sampson HA. *In silico* prediction of Ara h 2 T cell epitopes in peanut-allergic children. Clinical & Experimental Allergy. 2012;**43**:116-127. DOI: 10.1111/cea.12014

[77] Chen H, Yang H-W, Wei JF, Tao A-L. *In silico* prediction of the T-cell and IgE-binding epitopes of Per a 6 and Bla g 6 allergens in cockroaches. Molecular Medicine Reports. 2014;**10**:2130-2136. DOI: 10.3892/mmr.2014.2399

[78] Yang H, Chen H, Jin M, Xie H, He S, Wei J-F. Molecular cloning, expression, IgE binding activities and *in silico* epitope prediction of Per a 9 allergens of the American cockroach. International Journal of Molecular Sciences. 2016;**38**:1795-1805. DOI: 10.3892/ijmm.2016.2793

[79] Tong X, Guo M, Jin M, Chen H, Li Y, Wei J-F. *In silico* epitope prediction, expression and functional analysis of Per a 10 allergen from the American cockroach. International Journal of Molecular Sciences. 2016;**38**:1806-1814. DOI: 10.3892/ijmm.2016.2790

[80] Vormehr M, Schrörs B, Boegel S, Löwer M, Türeci Ö, Sahin U. Mutanome engineered RNA immunotherapy: Towards patient-centered tumor vaccination. Journal of Immunology Research. 2015;**2015**:1-6. DOI: 10.1155/2015/595363

[81] Castle JC, Kreiter S, Diekmann J, Löwer M, Roemer NVD, Graaf JD, Selmi A, Diken M, Boegel S, Paret C, Koslowski M, Kuhn AN, Britten CM, Huber C, Türeci Ö, Sahin U. Exploiting the mutanome for tumor vaccination. Cancer Research. 2012;**72**(5):1081-1091. DOI: 10.1158/0008-5472.CAN-11-3722

[82] Gfeller D, Bassani-Sternberg M, Schmidt J, Luescher IF. Current tools for predicting cancer-specific T cell immunity. Oncoimmunology. 2016;**5**(7):e1177691-1e1177691-9. DOI: 10.1080/2162402X.2016.1177691

[83] Mahdavi M, Moreau V. *In silico* designing breast cancer peptide vaccine for binding to MHC class I and II: A molecular docking study. Computational Biology and Chemistry. 2016;**65**:110-116. DOI: 10.1016/j.compbiolchem.2016.10.007

Section 6

Resolving Pertussis Resurgence

Chapter 8

Immunization against Pertussis: An Almost Solved Problem or a Headache in Public Health

Waldely de Oliveira Dias, Ana Fabíola R.O. Prestes, Priscila S. Cunegundes, Eliane P. Silva and Isaias Raw

Additional information is available at the end of the chapter

http://dx.doi.org/10.5772/intechopen.69283

Abstract

Whooping cough or pertussis is a serious infectious disease of the human respiratory tract, caused by Gram-negative bacteria *Bordetella pertussis* and *Bordetella parapertussis*$_{HU}$. The current pertussis vaccines may consist of dead cells of *B. pertussis* (whole cell pertussis vaccines—wPs) or purified antigens from the bacterium (acellular pertussis vaccines—aPs). The aPs are less reactogenic and have been widely used in developed countries for more than two decades, but their high cost of production makes them prohibitive for developing countries, and the accelerated rate of epidemic outbreaks has led to the hypothesis that aPs are less effective than the wP ones. Considering cost-effectiveness, some authors have pointed out questions about the possibility of reintroduction of wP vaccines into the primary doses of pertussis vaccination. The Butantan Institute in São Paulo, Brazil, developed a wP vaccine with low endotoxicity (Plow) obtained by chemical extraction of the lipooligosaccharide (LOS) fraction from the outer membrane of the bacterial cell, showing to be less reactogenic and equally immunogenic and protective as the traditional wP vaccine. The Plow may possibly be introduced into the vaccination schedule for immunization of adolescents and young adults in Brazil, an important epidemiological contribution to reducing the circulation of *B. pertussis*.

Keywords: pertussis, *Bordetella pertussis*, whole cell pertussis vaccine, acellular pertussis vaccine, resurgence of pertussis

1. Introduction

Pertussis or whooping cough is an acute and serious infectious disease of the respiratory tract, directly transmitted from human to human through respiratory aerosols [1]. The World Health Organization (WHO) estimates the annual incidence of 16 million cases of pertussis, with 195,000 deaths per year, one of the main causes of mortality for vaccine-preventable diseases in children less than five years [2, 3]. The main causative agent is the Gram-negative bacterium *Bordetella pertussis*, but although *Bordetella parapertussis*$_{HU}$ leads to a milder disease [4, 5], it has also been associated with more severe episodes, such as pneumonia and bronchopneumonia in children, with possible lethal consequences [6, 7]. The disease is exclusively human, with characteristics that differentiate it from other respiratory diseases [8, 9] and was widely disseminated in pre-vaccine era, mainly affecting children from 1 to 9 years of age. [10]. There is evidence that *B. pertussis* and *B. parapertussis*$_{HU}$ were adapted to restricted niches of hosts, which possibly allowed a more effective infection [11–14]. Pertussis toxin (PT), considered the main virulence factor of *B. pertussis*, is not produced by *B. parapertussis*, where the PT gene is transcriptionally silent [5, 15], which could be a reason for the frequently milder symptoms following infection by *B. parapertussis* [4, 5, 16, 17].

The classical manifestations of pertussis are divided into three phases: catarrhal, paroxysmal, and convalescent [18], and are particularly serious in unprotected newborns and young infants (<1 year old), with bacteria disseminating into the lungs causing necrotizing bronchiolitis, intra-alveolar hemorrhage, and fibrinous edema. In the most severe cases, there is usually intense lymphocytosis, correlated with pulmonary hypertension, respiratory failure, and death [19]. Older children, adolescents, and adults can also be affected [20], and although in these age groups the clinical manifestations may vary from the classic symptoms to moderate or even absent cough [21], high rates of the bacteria have been found in this population [9], who act as reservoirs and can transmit the infection to at-risk groups, such as neonates and infants [22].

2. Pertussis vaccines: an almost solved problem?

The initial attempts to develop a vaccine against *B. pertussis* occurred in a completely empirical way, after the culture of this bacterium in the laboratory by Jules Bordet and Octave Gengou, of the Pasteur Institute in Brussels in 1906 [23]. The first effective pertussis vaccine was developed in the 1930s by Pearl Kendrick and Grace Eldering using killed whole *B. pertussis* cells [24]. The introduction of such whole cell pertussis vaccines (wPs) in the late 1940s, right after combined with the diphtheria and tetanus toxoids for the formulation of the triple bacterial vaccine (DTP) [25], greatly reduced the incidence of the disease [9], leading to its almost eradication in the early 1970s [10]. However, although effective, wPs were associated with undesirable side effects, which led to a decrease in the acceptance of these vaccines and the rapid increase of pertussis incidence in several countries [26, 27]. In Great Britain, by 1977, the vaccination coverage rate for pertussis fell from 77 to 33%, and up to 9%, in some districts [28]. In Japan, the government suspended pertussis vaccination in February 1975, due to widespread publicity of two deaths in children, allegedly related to the vaccine, leading to a whopping cough peak two years later, accounting for 13,000 reported cases and 40 deaths [29, 30]. The reactogenicity of wPs was extensively evaluated in DTP, and the pertussis component proved to be mainly responsible for the toxicity of these combined vaccines. Summarizing the findings from these analyses, some authors report a prospective study conducted in Los Angeles from January 1978 to December 1979 in children of 0–6 years old, involving 15,752 doses of DTP and 784 doses of DT. The children were evaluated for local and systemic reactions occurring within 48 hours of immunization. Overall, all local and systemic reactions were significantly more frequent in children who had taken DTP vaccine than DT. At the site of application, redness, swelling, and pain occurred in 37.4, 40.7, and 50.9%, respectively, in those receiving DTP, but only 7.6, 7.6, and 9.9%, respectively, in those who received DT. The percentage of these reactions in DTP vaccinated increased from the first to the fifth dose [9].

The global consequence of the refusal to accept the wP vaccines resulted in the development of the first acellular pertussis vaccine (aP), the Japanese vaccine of Sato et al. [31], containing purified antigens from the bacterium. As there was an ongoing pertussis epidemic at that time, DTaP vaccines were very rapidly developed in Japan and immediately incorporated into their vaccine calendar in 1981 [32, 33]. In the late 1990s, the wPs were gradually replaced by aPs in many developed countries [34]. Current aP vaccines contain 1–5 purified pertussis proteins: inactivated PT, filamentous hemagglutinin (FHA), pertactin (PRN), and fimbriae 2 and 3 [35].

Nowadays, DTP vaccines are available in various formulations, containing whole cell (wP) or acellular (aP) pertussis component combined with diphtheria toxoid (D/d) and tetanus toxoid (T) to produce either full-strength— diphtheria/tetanus/wP (DTwP) or aP (DTaP) vaccines—or reduced antigen-content (Tdap) vaccines, which are used for primary (DTwP or DTaP) or booster (Tdap) immunization. Whole cell pertussis vaccines are not indicated for individuals over seven years of age, and WHO only recommends formulations with lower concentrations of diphtheria toxoid and pertussis (Tdap and Td) in order to reduce their reactogenicity [36, 37]. More recently, DTP is presented as the basis for combined vaccines containing additional antigens added alone or in combinations, such as *Haemophilus influenzae* type b (Hib), hepatitis B, and inactivated poliovirus [38–43], allowing the administration of multiple vaccine antigens in a single injection, leading to the induction of simultaneous immunity for multiple diseases [44, 45]. These combined vaccines were approved by the World Health Organization's Expanded Program on Immunization (EPI) [46–48], which substantially reduced the number of injections required in the childhood vaccine schedule. Clinical studies using the DTPa-HBV-IPV/Hib hexavalent vaccine have shown that it is safe and effective [45, 49], and the incidence of local and systemic adverse reactions was comparable to those observed after administration of single vaccines or other DTaP-based vaccines [50–53], always less reactogenic than the combinations using whole cell pertussis vaccine (DTPw) [52].

3. Pertussis resurgence: a multifactorial problem

The preliminary clinical trials comparing DTaP with DTwP in the 1990s suggested comparable efficacy and immunogenicity [54–58]. However, more recent data have shown that the disease is not adequately controlled and outbreaks have occurred, even in countries with extensive vaccine coverage [59–61]. The reasons for the apparent ineffectiveness of current vaccines and vaccination programs in the control of infection and transmission are unclear, but there are likely to be a number of factors contributing to the short-lived immunity after vaccination [62–64]. DTaP vaccines were licensed and recommended as a booster in the USA in 1992 and introduced as primary immunization in newborns in 1997. Currently, even with 95% vaccine coverage in newborns and use of booster dose in adolescents, pertussis is the least immunopreventable disease, with the highest incidence rates already reported in the post-vaccination era [65]. Possible reasons for the resurgence of pertussis include a reduction in vaccine efficacy, with rapid waning immunity, improvement in the epidemiological surveillance and diagnostic methods, and genetic changes in the pathogen [66].

DTaP vaccination induces excellent, but not durable, immune response [67–69]. The higher antigenic load of the wPs may explain the epidemiological evidence that supports the longer lasting protection induced by these vaccines, in relation to the aPs. Potentially protective antigens may be absent or may be in insufficient quantity in the aP formulations, or may exhibit poor cross-match with antigens present in the circulating bacterial strains [70]. The immunity conferred by DTaP drops every year after the fifth dose, so that 5 years after the last dose the probability of a child vaccinated with this vaccine to acquire the disease is four to fifteen times greater than that after the initial doses [63, 64, 71, 72], and 80% of these children are no longer protected at the time of Tdap booster [73]. The efficacy conferred by Tdap was 75.3% in a pertussis outbreak in Wisconsin in 2012, falling after 2 years to 34.5% [74].

Differences between wP and aP vaccines, related to its antigenic load and presentation of antigens to antigen presenting cells, lead to a different balance of Th1/Th2/Th17 response. The role of Th1 and Th17 cells has been demonstrated in the protective immunity induced by *B. pertussis* infection or immunization with wP, and on the other hand, immunization with an aP vaccine administered with alum as adjuvant induced Th2 and Th17 cells, but poor Th1 response [75]. The multiple virulence factors of *B. pertussis*, many of them efficiently maintained in the wP vaccines, presuppose a better stimulation of innate immunity, leading to the generation of effective Th1/Th17-skewed adaptive immunity [76].

The probability of contracting the disease of humans primed with DTwP is lower than those primed with DTaP [62, 63, 68, 69]. Adolescents vaccinated with three doses of DTaP were 3.3 times more likely to contract pertussis than children vaccinated only with DTwP [46, 62]. These data were recently confirmed in baboons, an animal model that reproduces the characteristics of human infection [77–79]. Baboons immunized with DTaP and challenged with a clinical isolate of *B. pertussis* are heavily colonized and do not control the infection until 4–5 weeks, transmitting the bacteria to naive animals. Those vaccinated with DTwP are colonized, but without leukocytosis, and control the infection in 2–3 weeks, faster than those not previously vaccinated [78].

There is evidence that circulating strains of *B. pertussis* are evolving to evade the vaccine-conferred immunity [80]. In fact, pertactin-deficient *B. pertussis* strains were identified in 85% of the isolates obtained from eight US states between 2011 and 2013 [81]. These samples emerged rapidly and did not express the PRN contained in the DTaP vaccine, and suggesting selective advantage, individuals previously vaccinated against pertussis had higher chance of infection with the PRN-deficient strains than with the strain expressing that protein [82–85]. Besides that, an increase in the incidence of vaccine alleles of *B. pertussis* could also suggest an evolutionary epitope-mediated vaccine pressure [86–89], contributing to the reemergence of pertussis in humans, and in this sense, it is also not clear how the *B. parapertussis* can answer to the selective pressure exerted by large-scale vaccination against *B. pertussis*.

Although highly effective in reducing the incidence of pertussis infections, the acellular pertussis vaccines have little or no efficacy against *B. parapertussis* [17, 90, 91]. Some authors have postulated that vaccination with aPs can interfere with the "clearance" of *B. parapertussis*, facilitating the adaptive performance of this pathogen, which could lead to the emergence of more susceptible hosts to *B. parapertussis* infection [92]. Accordingly, a gradual increase in the prevalence of *B. parapertussis* has been observed as a result of epidemiological pertussis immunization with vaccines that are less protective against *B. parapertussis* than the natural infection with *B. pertussis* [93]. Similar to the serum specificity observed in other infectious diseases, pertussis vaccines may have led to epidemiological pressure, with an increase in the prevalence of *B. parapertussis*. Since the differential diagnosis would not affect clinical procedures, the vast majority of pertussis studies are not directed to the identification of *B. parapertussis*, which probably has led to unreported cases. However, studies aimed at the differential diagnosis showed that *B. parapertussis* comprise from 2 to 36% of the cases [94].

In August 2015, the World Health Organization published its position on pertussis vaccines [95], in an attempt to provide substantiated information for immunization and public health programs, in a document that replaces the previous one published in 2010 [35]. The main goal of this position paper was to guide the choice of pertussis vaccines—wP or aP—to the most current strategies to reduce the risk of pertussis in infants and young children. In this document, it was established that the goal to be achieved in all countries is the maintenance of high vaccination coverage (higher than 90%). High levels of safety and protection can be obtained by the wP and the aP vaccines, after the primary series of immunization with three doses, ideally completed by the sixth month of life (**Table 1**). However, although systemic and local reactions are more commonly associated with wP, the duration of protection conferred by these vaccines is longer [96–98]. The pertussis vaccination schedule should maintain protection for at least six years in countries using wP, but the protection may suffer a marked decline before the age of six years when aP is used (**Table 1**) [95]. Vaccination of pregnant women has been recommended by WHO as the best strategy for disease prevention in infants too young to be vaccinated or with incomplete immunization schedule, and the change from wP to aP in primary immunization should only be considered in countries that are able to maintain a schedule with periodic reinforcement and sustainable maternal immunization. If this is not the case, immunization with wP should be maintained and in national programs using aP, consideration should be given to the introduction of additional booster doses in the case of pertussis reemergence [95]. The production cost of the aP vaccine is considerably higher than that of the wP (difference of more than 5 US$ per dose with PAHO's revolving

Balance of benefits and costs	Acellular pertussis vaccine (aP)	Whole cell pertussis vaccine (wP)
Quality of evidence for benefits	Highly effective	Highly effective
Intervention effects	• Primary series reduces the risk of severe pertussis • Lower incidence of adverse reactions than with wP vaccine [96, 97]	• Primary series reduces the risk of severe pertussis • Primary series not associated with serious adverse effects
Duration of protection	• May decline before 6 years	• At least 6 years • Longer than that induced by aP [98]
Resource implications	• Significantly more expensive than the wP vaccine	• Significantly less expensive than the aP vaccine

Table 1. WHO evidences to pertussis vaccines [95].

fund price), which has a direct implication in health systems, especially in underdeveloped and developing countries.

Considering cost-effectiveness in the implementation of national vaccination programs, some authors have pointed out questions about the possibility of reintroduction of wP vaccines into the primary doses of pertussis vaccination [76, 99, 100], which could again lead to the problems with the reactogenicity of these vaccines.

4. Back to the past: whole cell pertussis vaccine as a new alternative

In Brazil, mandatory notification of all outbreaks began in 1975 when the pertussis entered the list of notifiable diseases. In the early 1980s, more than 40,000 cases were reported per year, with an incidence rate >30/100,000 inhabitants. With the introduction of the DTP vaccine in the Brazilian scheme of childhood vaccination in 1983, this number fell sharply [101]. In 2002, the first three doses of the DTwP were replaced by the tetravalent vaccine DTwP + *H. influenzae* type B (DTwP-Hib), that in 2012 was replaced by the pentavalent DTwP + *H. influenzae* type B + hepatitis B (DTwP-Hib-HBV). The first three doses of the pentavalent vaccine are administered at 2, 4, and 6 months of age, followed by DTwP booster at 15 and 48 months of age. DTaP vaccine is recommended for children at increased risk of developing or who have developed severe adverse events to the DTwP, and the vaccine is available at the Special Immunobiological Reference Centers. After 2014 the Brazilian National Immunization Program began to offer Tdap to pregnant women [102]. Despite the high vaccination coverage (>95%) since 2011, a significant increase in the number of reported cases of pertussis in Brazil has been observed, with an incidence rate in 2013 of 14,058 confirmed cases/100,000 in infants under one year of age, the majority of cases and deaths in unvaccinated children younger than 4 months old [103].

The Butantan Institute in São Paulo, Brazil, produces DTwP vaccine since 1953. Currently, more than 90% of Brazilian children are vaccinated at the age of 2/4/6 and 15 months life,

http://dx.doi.org/10.5772/intechopen.69283

which are about 250 million doses annually. Over the past 20 years, the Institute has been investigating new pertussis vaccines, less reactogenic and at low cost [104].

Although effective, wP vaccines contain a significant amount of lipooligosaccharide (LOS), an endotoxin of Gram-negative outer membrane that may be involved in the local and systemic adverse vaccine reactions. The introduction of procedures that increase the safety of wP vaccines maintaining its effectiveness remains a very important aspect, especially for developing countries that do not have access to currently available aP vaccines. In this sense, a whole cell pertussis vaccine was developed with low endotoxicity (Plow) obtained by chemical extraction of the LOS fraction from the outer membrane of the bacterial cell [105]. This vaccine was evaluated as DTwP vaccine, combined with tetanus and diphtheria toxoids in a Phase I field trial in infants, showing to be less reactogenic and equally immunogenic and protective as the traditional DTP vaccine [106].

Many developed countries using acellular pertussis vaccines in infancy have introduced a booster dose for adolescents [107], preventing the carrier state, an attempt to block the spread of the disease to infants not immunized or with incomplete immunization schedule. Due to its low reactogenicity, the Plow vaccine may possibly be introduced into the vaccination schedule for immunization of adolescents and young adults in Brazil, an important epidemiological contribution to reducing the circulation of *B. pertussis*.

Preliminary studies in our laboratory have shown that the Plow is able to protect mice against *B. parapertussis* (unpublished data), suggesting an important role in the control of this pathogen, which has not been reached by vaccination with acellular pertussis vaccines [17, 90, 91, 108, 109].

The cost to produce the Plow vaccine is the same as the conventional whole cell pertussis vaccine, which makes its use feasible in developing countries, such as Brazil [89, 110], as an alternative for use in different strategies for the control of pertussis resurgence, including vaccination of adolescents and adults, due to their lower reactogenicity.

Acknowledgements

This work was funded by the Brazilian National Bank for Economic and Social Development (BNDES), National Council for Scientific and Technological Development (CNPq), and Butantan Foundation.

Author details

Waldely de Oliveira Dias*, Ana Fabíola R.O. Prestes, Priscila S. Cunegundes, Eliane P. Silva and Isaias Raw

*Address all correspondence to: waldely.dias@butantan.gov.br

Special Laboratory of Vaccine Development, Butantan Institute, São Paulo, Brazil

References

[1] de Greeff SC, Mooi FR, Westerhof A, Verbakel JM, Peeters MF, Heuvelman CJ, Notermans DW, Elvers LH, Schellekens JF, de Melker HE. Pertussis disease burden in the household: How to protect young infants. Clinical Infectious Diseases. 2010;**50**(10):1339-1345. DOI: 10.1086/652281

[2] Centers for Disease Control and Prevention. Pertussis. (Whooping Cough). 2016. Available from: https://www.cdc.gov/pertussis/countries/ [Accessed: March 28, 2017]

[3] Provisional 2015 Reports of Notifiable Diseases, January 8, 2016/64(52). Center for Disease Control and Prevention. Available from: http://www.cdc.gov/mmwr/preview/mmwrhtml/mm6452md.htm?s_cid=mm6452md_w [Accessed: March 28, 2017]

[4] Mastrantonio P, Stefanelli P, Giuliano M, Herrera Rojas Y, Ciofi degli Atti M, Anemona A, Tozzi AE. *Bordetella parapertussis* infection in children: Epidemiology, clinical symptoms, and molecular characteristics of isolates. Journal of Clinical Microbiology. 1998;**36**(4):999-1002

[5] Bergfors E, Trollfors B, Taranger J, Lagergard T, Sundh V, Zackrisson G. Parapertussis and pertussis: Differences and similarities in incidence, clinical course, and antibody responses. International Journal of Infectious Diseases. 1999;**3**:140-146. DOI: 10.1016/S1201-9712(99)90035-8

[6] Bjornstad ON, Harvill ET. Evolution and emergence of *Bordetella* in humans. Trends in Microbiology. 2005;**13**:355-359. DOI: 10.1016/j.tim.2005.06.007

[7] Preston A, Parkhill J, Maskell DJ. The Bordetellae: Lessons from genomics. Nature Reviews Microbiology. 2004;**2**:379-390. DOI: 10.1038/nrmicro886

[8] Cherry JD, Heininger U. Pertussis and other Bordetella infections. In: Feigin RD, Cherry JD, Demmler-Harrison GJ, Kaplan S, editors. Feigin and Cherry's Textbook of Pediatric Infectious Diseases. 6th ed. Philadelphia, PA: Elsevier Saunders; 2009. pp. 1683-1706

[9] Mattoo S, Cherry JD. Molecular pathogenesis, epidemiology, and clinical manifestations of respiratory infections due to Bordetella pertussis and other Bordetella subspecies. Clinical Microbiology Reviews. 2005;**18**:326-382. DOI: 10.1128/CMR.18.2.326-382.2005

[10] Centers for Disease Control and Prevention. Pertussis. In: Atkinson W, Wolfe S, Hamborsky J, editors. Epidemiology and Prevention of Vaccine-Preventable Diseases. 12th ed., second printing. Washington DC: Public Health Foundation; 2012. pp. 215-232

[11] Parkhill J, Sebaihia M, Preston A, et al. Comparative analysis of the genome sequences of *Bordetella pertussis, Bordetella parapertussis* and *Bordetella bronchiseptica*. Nature Genetics. 2003;**35**:32-40. DOI: 10.1038/ng1227

[12] Cummings CA, Brinig MM, Lepp PW, van de Pas S, Relman DA. *Bordetella* species are distinguished by patterns of substantial gene loss and host adaptation. Journal of Bacteriology. 2004;**186**:1484-1492. DOI: 10.1128/JB.186.5.1484-1492.2004

[13] Li LJ, Dougan G, Novotny P, Charles IG. P.70 pertactin, an outer-membrane protein from *Bordetella parapertussis*: Cloning, nucleotide sequence and surface expression in *Escherichia coli*. Molecular Microbiology. 1991;**5**:409-417. DOI: 10.1111/j.1365-2958.1991.tb02123.x

[14] Blom J, Hansen GA, Poulsen FM. Morphology of cells and hemagglutinogens of *Bordetella* species: Resolution of substructural units in fimbriae of *Bordetella pertussis*. Infection and Immunity. 1983;**42**:308-317

[15] Arico B, Rappuoli R. *Bordetella parapertussis* and *Bordetella bronchiseptica* contain transcriptionally silent pertussis toxin genes. Journal of Bacteriology. 1987;**169**:2847-2853. DOI: 10.1128/jb.169.6.2847-2853.1987

[16] Heininger U, Stehr K, Schmitt-Grohé S, Lorenz C, Rost R, Christenson PD, Uberall M, Cherry JD. Clinical characteristics of illness caused by *Bordetella parapertussis* compared with illness caused by *Bordetella pertussis*. Pediatric Infectious Disease Journal. 1994;**13**(4):306-309. DOI: 10.1097/00006454-199404000-00011

[17] Liese JG, Renner C, Stojanov S, Belohradsky BH. Clinical and epidemiological picture of *B pertussis* and *B parapertussis* infections after introduction of acellular pertussis vaccines. Archives of Disease in Childhood. 2003;**88**:684-687. DOI: 10.1136/adc.88.8.684

[18] American Academy of Pediatrics. Summaries of infectious diseases. In: Pickering LK, Baker J, Kimberlin DW, Long SS, editors. Red Book: 2012 Report of the Committee on Infectious Diseases. 29th ed. By: AAP Committee on Infectious Diseases. Elk Grove Village, IL; 2012. pp. 553-566

[19] Paddock CD, Sanden GN, Cherry JD, Gal AA, Langston C, Tatti KM, Wu KH, Goldsmith CS, Greer PW, Montague JL, Eliason MT, Holman RC, Guarner J, Shieh WJ, Zaki SR. Pathology and pathogenesis of fatal Bordetella pertussis infection in infants. Clinical Infectious Diseases. 2008;**47**(3):328-338. DOI: 10.1086/589753

[20] Nennig ME, Shinefield HR, Edwards KM, Black SB, Fireman BH. Prevalence and incidence of adult pertussis in an urban-population. Journal of the American Medical Association. 1996;**275**:1672-1674. DOI: 10.1001/jama.1996.03530450062034

[21] Ward JI, Cherry JD, Chang SJ, Partridge S, Keitel W, Edwards K, Lee M, Treanor J, Greenberg DP, Barenkamp S, Bernstein DI, Edelman R, APERT Study Group. Bordetella pertussis infections in vaccinated and unvaccinated adolescents and adults, as assessed in a national prospective randomized acellular pertussis vaccine trial. Clinical Infectious Diseases. 2006;**43**(2):151-157. DOI: 10.1086/504803

[22] Lavine J, Broutin H, Harvill ET, Bjornstad ON. Imperfect vaccine-induced immunity and whooping cough transmission to infants. Vaccine. 2010;**29**:11-16. DOI: 10.1016/j.vaccine.2010.10.029

[23] Bordet J, Gengou O. Le microbe de la coqueluche. Annales de l'Institut Pasteur. 1906;**2**:731-741

[24] Kendrick P, Eldering GA. A study in active immunization against pertussis. With statistical analyses of the data by AJ BOROWSKI. American Journal of Epidemiology. 1939;**29**:133-153. DOI: 10.1093/oxfordjournals.aje.a118485

[25] McIntyre P. Vaccination strategies for the prevention of neonatal pertussis. Expert Review of Vaccines. 2004;**34**:375-378. DOI: 10.1586/14760584.3.4.375

[26] Centers for Disease Control. International notes pertussis – England and Wales. Morbidity and Mortality Weekly Report. 1982;**31**(47): 629-640

[27] Baker JP. The pertussis vaccine controversy in Great Britain, 1974-1986. Vaccine. 2003;**21**:4003-4010. DOI: 10.1016/S0264-410X(03)00302-5

[28] Swansea Research Unit of the Royal College of General Practitioners. Effect of a low pertussis vaccination uptake on a large community. British Medical Journal. 1981;**282**(6268):23-26. DOI: 10.1136/bmj.282.6257.23

[29] Kanai K. Japan's experience in pertussis epidemiology and vaccination in the past thirty years. Japanese Journal of Medical Science and Biology. 1980;**33**:107-143. DOI: 10.7883/yoken1952.33.107

[30] Kimura M, Kuno-Sakai H. Pertussis vaccines in Japan—a clue toward understanding Japanese attitude to vaccines. Journal of Tropical Pediatrics. 1991;**37**:45-47. DOI: 10.1093/tropej/37.1.45

[31] Sato Y, Kimura M, Fukumi H. Development of a pertussis component vaccine in Japan. Lancet. 1984;**1**:122-126. DOI:.10.1016/S0140-6736(84)90061-8

[32] Kimura M, Kuno-Sakai H. Pertussis vaccines in Japan. Acta Paediatrica Japonica. 1988;**30**:143-153. DOI: 10.1111/j.1442-200X.1988.tb02512.x

[33] Noble GR, Bernier RH, Esber EC, Hardegree MC, Hinman AR, Klein D, Saah AJ. Acellular and whole-cell pertussis vaccines in Japan. Report of a visit by US scientists. Journal of the American Medical Association. 1987;**257**:1351-1356. DOI: 10.1001/jama.1987.03390100089032

[34] Preston A, Maskell DJ. A new era of research into Bordetella pertussis pathogenesis. Journal of Infection. 2002;**44**:13-16. DOI: 10.1053/jinf.2001.0933

[35] World Health Organization. Pertussis vaccines: WHO position paper. Weekly Epidemiological Record. 2010;**85**:385-400

[36] WHO. DTP Vaccine Rates Information Sheet. May 2014. Available from: http://www.who.int/vaccine_safety/initiative/tools/DTP_vaccine_rates_information_sheet.pdf [Accessed: March 28, 2017]

[37] WHO Report. Pertussis vaccines: WHO position paper, August 2015—Recommendations. Vaccine. 2016;**34**:1423-1425. DOI: 10.1016/j.vaccine.2015.10.136

[38] Committee on Infectious Diseases, American Academy of Pediatrics. Prevention of poliomyelitis: Recommendations for use of only inactivated poliovirus vaccine for routine immunization. Pediatrics. 1999;**104**:1404-1406

[39] Van Damme P. Hepatitis B: Vaccination programmes in Europe – An update. Vaccine. 2001;**19**:2375-2379. DOI: 10.1016/S0264-410X(00)00457-6

[40] Zepp F, Schuind A, Meyer C, S¨anger R, Kaufhold A, Willems P. Safety and reactogenicity of a novel DTPa-HBV-IPV combined vaccine given along with commercial Hib vaccines in comparison with separate concomitant administration of DTPa, Hib, and OPV vaccines in infants. Pediatrics. 2002;**109**:1-8

[41] Gylca R, Gylca V, Benes O, Melnic A, Chicu V, Weisbecker C, Willems P, Kaufhold A. A new DTPa-HBV-IPV vaccine co-administered with Hib, compared to a commercially available DTPw-IPV/Hib vaccine co-administered with HBV, given at 6, 10 and 14 weeks following HBV at birth. Vaccine. 2000;**19**:825-833. DOI: 10.1016/S0264-410X(00)00231-0

[42] Decker MD, Edwards KM, Steinhoff MC, Rennels MB, Pichichero ME, Englund JA, Anderson EL, Deloria MA, Reed GF. Comparison of 13 acellular pertussis vaccines: Adverse reactions. Pediatrics. 1995;**96**:557-566

[43] Yeh SH, Ward JI, Partridge S, Marcy SM, Lee H, Jing J, et al. Safety and immunogenicity of a pentavalent diphtheria, tetanus, pertussis, hepatitis B and polio combination vaccine in infants. Pediatric Infectious Disease Journal. 2001;**20**:973-980

[44] Andre FE. Development and clinical application of new polyvalent combined paediatric vaccines. Vaccine. 1999;**17**:1620-1627. DOI: 10.1016/S0264-410X(98)00426-5

[45] Dodd D. Benefits of combination vaccines: Effective vaccination on a simplified schedule. American Journal of Managed Care. 2003;**9**(Suppl.):S6-S12

[46] Report of the Global Advisory Group. Expanded Programme on Immunization. Weekly Epidemiological Record. 1992;**67**:11-15

[47] WHO. Hepatitis B vaccine-making global progress. Expanded Programme on Immunization. WHO Update; 1996

[48] Global Programme for Vaccine and Immunization (GPV). The WHO position paper on *Haemophilus influenzae* type b conjugate vaccines. Weekly Epidemiological Record. 1998;**73**:64-68

[49] Capiau C, Poolman J, Hoet B, Bogaerts H, Andre F. Development and clinical testing of multivalent vaccines based on a diphtheria-tetanus acellular pertussis vaccine: Difficulties encountered and lessons learned. Vaccine. 2003;**21**:2273-2287. DOI: 10.1016/S0264-410X(03)00107-5

[50] Zepp F, Knuf M, Heininger U, Jahn K, Collard A, Habermehl P, et al. Safety, reactogenicity and immunogenicity of a combined hexavalent tetanus, diphtheria, acellular pertussis, hepatitis B, inactivated poliovirus vaccine and *Haemophilus influenzae* type b conjugate vaccine, for primary immunization of infants. Vaccine. 2004;**22**:2226-2233. DOI: 10.1016/j.vaccine.2003.11.044

[51] Saenger R, Maechler G, Potreck M, Zepp F, Knuf M, Habermehl P, et al. Booster vaccination with hexavalent DTPa-HBV-IPV/Hib vaccine in the second year of life is as safe as concomitant DTPa-IPV/Hib+HBV administered separately. Vaccine. 2005;**23**:1135-1143. DOI: 10.1016/j.vaccine.2004.08.030

[52] Cohen R, Schuerman L. Reactogenicity of a new DTPa-HBV-IPV (+ and /Hib) vaccines after primary and booster doses. Presented at: 18th Annual Meeting of the European Society for Pediatric Infectious Diseases (ESPID) Noordwijk, The Netherlands, 2000

[53] *Infanrix hexa*TM. Product Monograph. GlaxoSmithKline; 2016 GlaxoSmithKline Inc. 7333 Mississauga Road Mississauga, Ontario L5N 6L4

[54] Lugauer S, Heininger U, Cherry JD, Stehr K. Long-term clinical effectiveness of an acellular pertussis component vaccine and a whole cell pertussis component vaccine. European Journal of Pediatrics. 2002;**161**:142-146. DOI: 10.1007/s00431-001-0893-5

[55] Salmaso S, Mastrantonio P, Tozzi AE, Stefanelli P, Anemona A, Ciofi degli Atti ML, Giammanco A, Group SIW. Sustained efficacy during the first 6 years of life of 3-component acellular pertussis vaccines administered in infancy: The Italian experience. Pediatrics. 2001;**108**:E81. DOI: 10.1542/peds.108.5.e81

[56] Taranger J, Trollfors B, Lagergård T, Lind L, Sundh V, Zackrisson G, Bryla DA, Robbins JB. Unchanged efficacy of a pertussis toxoid vaccine throughout the two years after the third vaccination of infants. Pediatric Infectious Disease Journal. 1997;**16**(2):180-184. DOI: 10.1097/00006454-199702000-00003

[57] Edwards KM, Decker MD. Pertussis vaccines. In: Plotkin SA, Orenstein WA, Offit PA, editors. Vaccines. 6th ed. Edinburgh, Scotland: Elsevier Saunders; 2013. pp. 447-492

[58] Plotkin SA, Cadoz M. The acellular pertussis vaccine trials: An interpretation. Pediatric Infectious Disease Journal. 1997;**16**:508-517. DOI: 10.1097/00006454-199705000-00011

[59] Cherry JD. Epidemic pertussis in 2012 – The resurgence of a vaccine preventable disease. New England Journal of Medicine. 2012;**367**:785-787. DOI: 10.1056/NEJMp1209051

[60] Chiappini E, Stival A, Galli L, de Martino M. Pertussis re-emergence in the post-vaccination era. BMC Infectious Diseases. 2013;**13**:151. DOI: 10.1186/1471-2334-13-151

[61] Clark TA, Messionier NE, Hadler SC. Pertussis control: Time for something new? Trends in Microbiology. 2012;**20**:211-213. DOI: 10.1016/j.tim.2012.03.003

[62] Sheridan SL, Ware RS, Grimwood K, Lambert SB. Number and order of whole cell pertussis vaccines in infancy and disease protection. Journal of the American Medical Association. 2012;**308**:454-456. DOI: 10.1001/jama.2012.6364

[63] Klein NP, Bartlett J, Rowhani-Rahbar A, Fireman B, Baxter R. Waning protection after fifth dose of acellular pertussis vaccine in children. New England Journal of Medicine. 2012;**367**:1012-1019. DOI: 10.1056/NEJMoa1200850

[64] Misegades LK, Winter K, Harriman K, Talarico J, Messonnier NE, Clark TA, Martin SW. Association of childhood pertussis with receipt of 5 doses of pertussis vaccine by time since last vaccine dose, California, 2010. Journal of the American Medical Association. 2012;**308**(20):2126-2132. DOI: 10.1001/jama.2012.14939

[65] Centers for Disease Control and Prevention. Notifiable diseases and mortality tables. Morbidity and Mortality Weekly Report. 2013;**62**:669-682. Available from: https://www.cdc.gov/mmwr/volumes/65/wr/mm6522md.htm [Accessed: March 28, 2017]

[66] Cherry JD. Pertussis: Challenges today and for the future. PLoS Pathogens. 2013;**9**(7):e1003418. DOI: 10.1371/journal.ppat.1003418

[67] Warfel JM, Edwards KM. Pertussis vaccines and the challenge of inducing durable immunity. Current Opinion in Immunology. 2015;**35**:48-54. DOI: 10.1016/j.coi.2015.05.008

[68] Witt MA, Arias L, Katz PH, Truong ET, Witt DJ. Reduced risk of pertussis among persons ever vaccinated with whole cell pertussis vaccine compared to recipients of acellular pertussis vaccines in a large US cohort. Clinical Infectious Diseases. 2013;**56**:1248-1254. DOI: 10.1093/cid/cit046

[69] Liko J, Robison SG, Cieslak PR. Priming with whole-cell versus acellular pertussis vaccine. New England Journal of Medicine. 2013;**368**:581-582. DOI: 10.1056/NEJMc1212006

[70] Mooi FR, Van Der Maas NA, De Melker HE. Pertussis resurgence: Waning immunity and pathogen adaptation: Two sides of the same coin. Epidemiology and Infection. 2013;**13**:1-10. DOI: 10.1017/S0950268813000071

[71] Tartof SY, Lewis M, Kenyon C, White K, Osborn A, Liko J, Zell E, Martin S, Messonnier NE, Clark TA, Skoff TH. Waning immunity to pertussis following 5 doses of DTaP. Pediatrics. 2013;**131**(4):e1047-e1052. DOI: 10.1542/peds.2012-1928

[72] Witt MA, Katz PH, Witt DJ. Unexpectedly limited durability of immunity following acellular pertussis vaccination in preadolescents in a North American outbreak. Clinical Infectious Diseases. 2012;**54**:1730-1735. DOI: 10.1093/cid/cis287

[73] McGirr A, Fisman DN. Duration of pertussis immunity after DTaP immunization: A meta-analysis. Pediatrics. 2015;**135**:331-343. DOI: 10.1542/peds.2014-1729

[74] Koepke R, Eickhoff JC, Ayele RA, Petit AB, Schauer SL, Hopfensperger DJ, Conway JH, Davis JP. Estimating the effectiveness of tetanus-diphtheria-acellular pertussis vaccine (Tdap) for preventing pertussis: Evidence of rapidly waning immunity and difference in effectiveness by Tdap brand. Journal of Infectious Diseases. 2014;**210**:942-953. DOI: 10.1093/infdis/jiu322

[75] Ross PJ, Sutton CE, Higgins S, Allen AC, Walsh K, Misiak A, Lavelle EC, McLoughlin RM, Mills KH. Relative contribution of Th1 and Th17 cells in adaptive immunity to Bordetella pertussis: Towards the rational design of an improved acellular pertussis vaccine. PLoS Pathogens. 2013;**9**(4):e1003264. DOI: 10.1371/journal.ppat.1003264

[76] Ausiello CM, Cassone A. Acellular pertussis vaccines and pertussis resurgence: Revise or replace? mBio. 2014;**5**(3):e01339-14. DOI: 10.1128/mBio.01339-14

[77] Warfel JM, Beren J, Kelly VK, Lee G, Merkel TJ. Nonhuman primate model of pertussis. Infection and Immunity. 2012;**80**:1530-1536. DOI: 10.1128/IAI.06310-11

[78] Warfel JM, Zimmerman LI, Merkel TJ. Acellular pertussis vaccines protect against disease but fail to prevent infection and transmission in a nonhuman primate model. Proceedings of the National Academy of Sciences of the United States of America. 2014;**111**:787-792. DOI: 10.1073/pnas.1314688110

[79] Warfel JM, Merkel TJ. Bordetella pertussis infection induces a mucosal IL-17 response and long-lived Th17 and Th1 immune memory cells in nonhuman primates. Mucosal Immunology. 2013;**6**(4):787-796. DOI: 10.1038/mi.2012.117

[80] Bart MJ, Harris SR, Advani A, Arakawa Y, Bottero D, Bouchez V, Cassiday PK, Chiang CS, Dalby T, Fry NK, et al. Global population structure and evolution of *Bordetella pertussis* and their relationship with vaccination. mBio. 2014;**5**(2):e01074-14. DOI: 10.1128/mBio.01074-14

[81] Martin SW, Pawloski L, Williams M, Weening K, DeBolt C, Qin X, Reynolds L, Kenyon C, Giambrone G, Kudish K, Miller L, Selvage D, Lee A, Skoff TH, Kamiya H, Cassiday PK, Tondella ML, Clark TA. Pertactin negative Bordetella pertussis strains: Evidence for a possible selective advantage. Clinical Infectious Diseases. 2015;**60**(2):223-227. DOI: 10.1093/cid/ciu788

[82] Pawloski LC, Queenan AM, Cassiday PK, Lynch AS, Harrison MJ, Shang W, Williams MM, Bowden KE, Burgos-Rivera B, Qin X, Messonnier N, Tondella ML. Prevalence and molecular characterization of pertactin deficient Bordetella pertussis in the United States. Clinical and Vaccine Immunology. 2014;**21**(2):119-125. DOI: 10.1128/CVI.00717-13

[83] Queenan AM, Cassiday PK, Evangelista A. Pertactin-negative variants of Bordetella pertussis in the United States. New England Journal of Medicine. 2013;**368**:583-584. DOI: 10.1056/NEJMc1209369

[84] Hegerle N, Guiso N. Bordetella pertussis and pertactin deficient clinical isolates: Lessons for pertussis vaccines. Expert Review of Vaccines. 2014;**13**:1135-1146. DOI: 10.1586/14760584.2014.932254

[85] Lam C, Octavia S, Ricafort L, Sintchenko V, Gilbert GL, Wood N, McIntyre P, Marshall H, Guiso N, Keil AD, Lawrence A, Robson J. Rapid increase in pertactin-deficient Bordetella pertussis isolates, Australia. Emerging Infectious Diseases. 2014;**20**:626-633. DOI: 10.3201/eid2004.131478

[86] Elomaa A, Advani A, Donnelly D, Antila M, Mertsola J, Hallander H, He Q. Strain variation among Bordetella pertussis isolates in Finland, where the whole cell pertussis vaccine has been used for 50 years. Journal of Clinical Microbiology. 2005;**43**:3681-3687. DOI: 10.1128/JCM.43.8.3681-3687.2005

[87] van Amersfoorth SC, Schouls LM, van der Heide HG, Advani A, Hallander HO, Bondeson K, von König CH, Riffelmann M, Vahrenholz C, Guiso N, Caro V, Njamkepo E, He Q, Mertsola J, Mooi FR. Analysis of Bordetella pertussis populations in European countries with different vaccination policies. Journal of Clinical Microbiology. 2005;**43:**2837-2843. DOI: 10.1128/JCM.43.6.2837-2843.2005

[88] van Gent M, de Greeff SC, van der Heide HG, Mooi FR. An investigation into the cause of the 1983 whooping cough epidemic in the Netherlands. Vaccine. 2009;**27**(13):1898-1903. DOI: 10.1016/j.vaccine.2009.01.111

[89] Berbers GA, de Greeff SC, Mooi FR. Improving pertussis vaccination. Human Vaccine. 2009;**5**:497-503. DOI: 10.4161/hv.8112

[90] Willems RJ, Kamerbeek J, Geuijen CA, Top J, Gielen H, Gaastra W, Mooi FR. The efficacy of a whole cell pertussis vaccine and fimbriae against *Bordetella pertussis* and *Bordetella parapertussis* infections in a respiratory mouse model. Vaccine. 1998;**16**:410-416. DOI: 10.1016/S0264-410X(97)80919-X

[91] David S, van Furth R, Mooi FR. Efficacies of whole cell and acellular pertussis vaccines against *Bordetella parapertussis* in a mouse model. Vaccine. 2004;**22**(15):1892-1898. DOI: 10.1016/j.vaccine.2003.11.005

[92] Long GH, Karanikas AT, Harvill ET, Read AF, Hudson PJ. Acellular pertussis vaccination facilitates *Bordetella parapertussis* infection in a rodent model of bordetellosis. Proceedings. Biological Sciences. 2010;**277**(1690):2017-2025. DOI: 10.1098/rspb.2010.0010

[93] Restif O, Wolfe DN, Goebel EM, Bjørnstad ON, Harvill ET. Of mice and men: Asymmetric interactions between *Bordetella* pathogen species. Parasitology. 2008;**135**:1517-1529. DOI: 10.1017/S0031182008000279

[94] Watanabe M, Nagai M. Whooping cough due to *Bordetella parapertussis*: An unresolved problem. Expert Review of Anti-infective Therapy. 2004;**2**:447-454. DOI: 10.1586/14787210.2.3.447

[95] World Health Organization. Pertussis vaccines: WHO position paper. Weekly Epidemiological Record. 2015;**90**:433-460. Available from: http://www.who.int/wer/2015/wer9035.pdf [Accessed: March 31, 2017]

[96] Jefferson T, Rudin M, DiPietrantonj C. Systematic review of the effects of pertussis vaccines in children. Vaccine. 2003;**21**:2003-2014. DOI: 10.1016/S0264-410X(02)00770-3

[97] Bar-On ES, Goldberg E, Hellmann S, Leibovici L. Combined DTP-HBV-HIB vaccine versus separately administered DTPHBV and HIB vaccines for primary prevention of diphtheria, tetanus, pertussis, hepatitis B and Haemophilus influenzae B (HIB). Cochrane Database of Systematic Reviews 2012, Issue 4. Art. No.: CD005530. DOI: 0.1002/14651858.CD005530.pub3

[98] Quinn HE, Mcintyre PB. Pertussis epidemiology in Australia over the decade 1995-2005, trends by region and age group. Communicable Diseases Intelligence. 2007;**31**(2):205-215

[99] Meade BD, Plotkin SA, Locht C. Possible options for new pertussis vaccines. The Journal of Infectious Diseases. 2014;**209**(S1):S24-S27. DOI: 10.1093/infdis/jit531

[100] Locht C, Mielcarek N. New pertussis vaccination approaches: En route to protect newborns? FEMS Immunology & Medical Microbiology. 2012;**66**:121-133. DOI: 10.1111/j.1574-695X.2012.00988.x

[101] Torres RSLA, Santos TZ, Torres RAA, Pereira VVG, Fávero LAF, Filho ORM, Penkal ML, Araujo LS. Resurgence of pertussis at the age of vaccination: Clinical, epidemiological, Wand molecular aspects. Jornal de Pediatria (Rio J). 2015;**91**(4):333-338. DOI: 10.1016/j.jped.2014.09.004

[102] Brazilian Ministry of Health. Informe Técnico para Implantação da Vacina Adsorvida Difteria, Tétano e Coqueluche (Pertussis Acelular) Tipo adulto – dTpa. 2014. Available from: http://www.crmpr.org.br/uploadAddress/info_dtpa_ministerio-saude-setembro-2014%5B1614%5D.pdf

[103] Guimarães LM, Carneiro ELNC, Carvalho-Costa FA. Increasing incidence of pertussis in Brazil: A retrospective study using surveillance data. BMC Infectious Diseases. 2015;**15**:442-453. DOI: 10.1186/s12879-015-1222-3

[104] Dias WO, Leite LCC, Horton DSPQ, Sakauchi MA, Kubrusly FS, Furuyama N, Nascimento IP, Quintilio W, Higashi HG, Raw I. New approaches in pertussis vaccines for developing countries. In: Méndez-Vilas A, editor. Communicating Current Research and Educational Topics and Trends in Applied Microbiology. FORMATEX C/ Zurbarán 1, 2º - Oficina 1 06002 Badajoz Spain Vol. 2. 2007.pp. 668-672

[105] Dias WO, van der Ark AAJ, Sakaushi MA, Kubrusly FS, Prestes AFRO, Borges MM, Furuyama N, Horton DSPQ, Quintilio W, Antoniazi M, Kyipers B, van der Zeijst BAM, Raw I. A whole cell pertussis with reduced content of endotoxin. Human Vaccines & Immunotherapeutics. 2013;**9**(2):339-348. DOI: 10.4161/hv.22847

[106] Zorzeto TQ, Higashi HG, da Silva MTN, Carniel EF, Dias WO, Ramalho VD, Mazzola TN, Lima SCBS, Morcillo AM, Stephano MA, Antonio MARG, Zanolli ML, Raw I, Vilela MMS. Immunogenicity of a whole-cell pertussis vaccine with low lipopolysaccharide content in infants. Clinical and Vaccine Immunology. 2009;**16**:544-550. DOI: 10.1128/CVI.00339-08

[107] Cornia PB, Hersh AL, Lipsky BA, Newman TB, Gonzales R. Does this coughing adolescent or adult patient have pertussis? Journal of the American Medical Association. 2010;**304**(8):890-896. DOI: 10.1001/jama.2010.1181

[108] Khelef N, Danve B, Quentin-Millet MJ, Guiso N. *Bordetella pertussis* and *Bordetella parapertussis*: Two immunologically distinct species. Infection and Immunity. 1993;**61** (2):486-490

[109] Stehr K, Cherry JD, Heininger U, Schmitt-Grohé S, Uberall M, Laussucq S, Eckhardt T, Meyer M, Engelhardt R, Christenson P. A comparative efficacy trial in Germany in infants who received either the Lederle/Takeda acellular pertussis component DTP (DTaP) vaccine, the Lederle whole-cell component DTP vaccine, or DT vaccine. Pediatrics. 1998;**101**(1):1-11

[110] Higashi HG, Luna E, Precioso AR, Vilela M, Kubrusly FS, Dias WO, Raw I. Acellular and "low" pertussis vaccines: Adverse events and the role of mutations. The Revista do Instituto de Medicina Tropical de São Paulo. 2009;**51**(3):131-134. DOI: 10.1590/S0036-46652009000300002

Section 7

Vaccine Side Effects

Chapter 9

Adverse Events Related to Vaccination (VAEs): How to Manage the Further Doses of Immunization and Parents' Hesitancy

Guido Castelli Gattinara, Elena Bellelli,
Donatella F. Angelone, Veronica Santilli and
Luciana Nicolosi

Additional information is available at the end of the chapter

http://dx.doi.org/10.5772/intechopen.68697

Abstract

This study supports the evidence that after vaccine-related reactions, it is still possible to carry out the immunization protocol.

Out of more than 1000 patients per year evaluated for potential vaccine-related risks (patients with chronic/serious diseases and events connected with vaccination), 76 (6%) presented previous vaccine adverse events (VAEs). The decision about whether to continue child vaccination is made evaluating different factors: absence of specific contraindications, parents' counseling, adequate hospital setting, choice of an appropriate and individualized schedule. None of the 76 children vaccinated after VAEs presented further side effects.

Our data demonstrate that VAE is not a recurring event. The real risk of a new VAE is mostly associated with the serious allergic reactions (IgE-mediated anaphylaxis) and parents should be aware of this information, so that the widespread fear of VAE recurrence can be contained. Indeed, this type of concerns represents one of the main reasons for vaccination hesitancy, which leads to incomplete vaccination schedules.

Conclusions: This chapter encourages clinicians to take advantage of the available VAE assessment algorithms to objectively evaluate real vaccine risk of VAE and provide parents with correct information, considering that VAEs are rare and severe reactions are extremely rare.

Keywords: vaccine, adverse event, side effect, re-vaccination, causality assessment, VAE

1. Introduction

A vaccine adverse event (VAE), also referred to as an adverse event following immunization, has been defined as "a medical incident that takes place after immunization, causes concern and is believed to be caused by the immunization" [1, 2]. These events are individual reactions usually induced by a direct effect of the vaccine or one of its components and are related with underlying medical conditions or idiosyncratic responses of the recipient. The adverse event may be any unfavorable or unintended sign, abnormal laboratory finding, symptom, or disease [3]. However, any untoward medical occurrence, which follows immunization and which does not necessarily have a causal relationship with the administration of the vaccine, is considered as VAE. These include also those conditions that would have occurred later on in life but are triggered earlier by the vaccination, like febrile seizures.

The adverse event may be a true adverse reaction that is induced by the vaccine, or may be caused by the way it is administered. Some events result from inappropriate practices, such as wrong dose, route, site or technique of administration, inappropriate intervals, incorrect preparation or amount of diluent, contamination, wrong storage, or ignored contraindications.

Other VAEs may be coincidental and would have occurred regardless of vaccination. These are purely temporally associated, because vaccines in children are given at an age when they are susceptible to many diseases. When a VAE is coincidental, the event would have occurred even if the individual had not been immunized. Sudden infant death syndrome (SIDS), for example, is an event clearly unrelated to vaccination; however, serious clinical events may be blamed to the vaccine by parents or community because of its close temporal association with immunization, especially if the vaccinated individual was previously healthy.

A vaccine safety surveillance program named Vaccine Adverse Event Reporting System (VAERS), run by the Center of Diseases Control and Prevention and Food and Drug Administration, has been instituted in 1990 in the US to collect information about VAEs [4]. In 1999, the World Health Organization (WHO) established the Global Advisory Committee of Vaccine Safety to respond promptly, efficiently, and with scientific rigor to vaccine safety issues of potential global importance. The last committee report edited on December 2015 is published and available online [5].

The main concern for both clinicians and people is to be able to distinguish between a real VAE and another health problem that is just temporally coincidental and not related to vaccination. This is particularly true in our era of vaccine skepticism: due to parents' frequent hesitation or outright refusal to accept some or all of the recommended vaccines, vaccination coverage is progressively decreasing [6]. The main reasons why people refuse vaccinations include ignorance about how vaccines work, which leads to an inappropriate criticism due to misunderstandings [7], and the negative influence by the media about vaccination safety and efficacy [8]. Whatever the cause, VAEs can upset people to the point of refusing further vaccination for their children [9].

To correctly interpret VAEs, the following characteristics need to be evaluated: the time correlation between vaccination and symptoms, the general health conditions of the subjects, and in particular their predisposition to allergies, and the known correlations between specific vaccines and clinical manifestations. In 2013, WHO edited the "User Manual for the revised classification on Causality assessment of adverse events following immunizations," a guide to a systematic and standardized causality assessment process for VAEs [10]. The manual suggests to adopt a systematic approach considering both the population (i.e., statistical strength of association between vaccine and VAE, biological plausibility, and coherence of the association) and the individual (i.e., relationship between vaccine and VAE, clinical and/or laboratory proof of the association, and exclusion of alternative explanations) levels. Recently, some authors have proposed other "causality assessment schemes" to help clinicians distinguish between VAEs whose association with the vaccination is consistent, indeterminate, or inconsistent [11].

1.1. Kinds of VAEs

The most typical and worrisome VAEs are allergic reactions, since reactions to the next dose of the same vaccine may be more immediate and severe than the first one, sometimes also life threatening [12]. Immediate allergic reactions are the most severe. These are relatively easy to identify because they are IgE-mediated and can be detected either by skin prick tests (SPTs) or *in vitro* by specific IgE assay [13]. One of the most serious VAEs is anaphylaxis, which could have life-threatening features: circulatory failure (altered level of consciousness, low blood pressure, weakness or absence of peripheral pulses, cold extremities due by reduced peripheral circulation, flushed face, and increased perspiration), with or without respiratory difficulties (bronchospasm and/or laryngospasm/laryngeal edema), normally with rapid onset (minutes), an unpredictable clinical course, and variable severity. Over 80–90% of anaphylaxis also presented skin and mucous membrane manifestations. Diagnosis of anaphylaxis is supported by the presence, following administration of a vaccine to a healthy recipient, of two or more of the above system signs and symptoms, which occur with a rapid onset. Anaphylactic reactions to vaccines are extremely rare but have the potential to be fatal.

It should be highlighted that the incidence of severe allergic reactions is very low, ranging between 0.5 and one cases/100,000 doses [14]. Currently, in Australia and US, anaphylaxis and encephalopathy are the only conditions determining absolute contraindication to revaccination with the suspect vaccine [15, 16]. Allergic children can also be at risk of reactions against non-active vaccine components, such as eggs/gelatin/antibiotics. Schemes with recommendations for vaccination of such allergic children have been developed [17].

A kind of VAEs that are particularly worrisome for parents is hypotonia-hyporesponsiveness episode (HHE), which is characterized by the sudden onset of pallor or cyanosis, decreased level or loss of responsiveness, and decreased level of muscle tone, occurring within 48 h of vaccination, normally transient and self-limiting. These episodes have been described to occur after vaccination with hexavalent vaccine and are considered to be related to the pertussis component [18]. A review of Canadian tertiary-care hospitals has shown that HHE accounts for less than five cases per 100,000 admissions to hospitalization, the majority of whom are discharged within 24 h [19]. Current evidences do not suggest that HHEs are associated with long-term morbidity or mortality.

Febrile seizures are among VAEs of particular parents' concern. However, febrile seizures are relatively common in children between 6 months and 5 years, and are more frequent in subjects with familiar and/or individual predisposition.

Other systemic reactions are fever, malaise, myalgia, irritability, headache, and loss of appetite. Inconsolable continuous crying lasting at least 3 h accompanied by high-pitched screaming can occur. The arthralgia usually including the small peripheral joints is infrequent but can be persistent lasting longer than 10 days. Rarely rubella vaccine can cause an acute arthropathy that lasts 10 days. Guillain-Barrè syndrome (GBS): acute onset of rapidly progressive, ascending, symmetrical flaccid paralysis, without fever and with sensory loss could occur after 30–60 days after immunization. Encephalopathy/encephalitis occurs within 72 h to 4 weeks after vaccination, as an acute onset of seizures or severe alternation in the level of consciousness and/or distinct change in behavior lasting 1 day or more. Idiopathic thrombocytopenic purpura (ITP) often follows measles vaccines. The timing and severity of these systemic reactions varies according to the characteristics of the vaccine received, the age of the recipient, and the individual biological response to each vaccine: it can start within a few hours to several days after vaccine.

A different kind of VAEs is represented by local reactions. These are frequently reported as "hypersensitivity reactions": pain, swelling, or redness at the site of injection usually starting within a few hours are generally mild and self-limiting. These are not allergic reactions, but may be due to a direct effect of the vaccine product, or be related to a higher antibody titers. Also, errors in vaccine preparation, in handling, or administration can cause local adverse effects, as purulence, inflammation, and positive Gram stain culture. Nodules at the injection site are relatively frequent and are constituted by a small well-defined mass or a lump at the injection site, which are indicated as a subcutaneous nodule, antigen cysts, or granulomas, in the absence of abscess formation, erythema, and warmth. Local reactions are generally of moderate entity but can be significant at times, making parents and patients antonyms to revaccination. Local reactions are commonly observed following tetanus, pertussis, and diphtheria vaccine: reports demonstrated that the rate and severity increase with booster compared with primary doses of these antigens [20–25].

Another event that often occurs after vaccination is fainting. It is considered a vasovagal response and usually takes place in older children and adolescents who are prone to this kind of reaction. It is not considered to be a serious reaction and never represents a contraindication to continue vaccination schedule. Canadians have proposed immunization guidelines on pain mitigation to help clinicians to prevent the aforementioned situations [26].

In our vaccine unit at the Bambino Gesù Pediatric Hospital in Rome, we visit about 1000 patients per year and we evaluate those who have one or more risk factors for vaccination.

About 6% of patients at risk for vaccination has a history of VAE. The decision on the opportunity to continue the vaccination schedule is made upon the evaluation of various factors. In case specific contraindications are not highlighted, we administer vaccines following a patient-individualized schedule.

Here, we present the results of the analysis of data on patients with history of VAEs that came to our attention between September 2014 and February 2016.

2. Materials and methods

We included in our analysis all children who have been vaccinated at the Vaccine Unit of Bambino Gesù Children Hospital from September 10, 2014, until February 18, 2016. On a total of 1367 enrolled subjects, 76 children (6%) came to our unit with a previous history of one or more VAEs. In case of more than one VAEs, these were classified as "main event" and "secondary event" depending on the severity of reported symptoms.

We recorded patients' familial and personal history, predisposition to allergies, time correlation between vaccine administration and VAE, severity of referred VAE (i.e., grade 1: mild; grade 2: moderate; grade 3: severe), if the previous VAE has caused hospitalization, VAE duration, and sequela of the previous VAE.

Based on this general evaluation, we decided whether patients could continue to be vaccinated or not. For those who were, we created a personalized vaccine schedule and provided them with a vaccination follow-up plan in our unit.

3. Results

3.1. Previous, referred VAE

Patients' characteristic: The median age of the 76 patients affected by a previous VAE was 3.9 ± 4 years.

VAEs type: The most common was urticaria/angioedema, which was referred by 31 out of 76 patients (41%). Other common VAEs were hypotonia/sleepiness (11 patients = 14%), local symptoms (7 patients = 9%), high fever (6 patients = 8%), and low fever (5 patients = 7%). In our sample, seizures were relatively rare (3 patients = 4%). Anaphylaxis, the most severe VAE, was referred only by 1 patient after hexavalent vaccine administration. Guillain-Barrè syndrome, another severe adverse event, was referred by 1 patient after mumps, measles, and rubella (MMR) vaccine (**Table 1**). Sixteen patients (21%) reported positive personal and/or familiar history regarding allergies. In all cases, the referred VAE was supposedly of allergic nature and the patient or his/her parents were allergic.

VAEs entity: The main referred VAE was classified as mild in 13 out of 76 patients (17%), moderate in 54 (71%), and severe in 9 (12%) patients. The mean time interval between vaccination

	N reported events	% on reported events[a]	% on observed patients[b]
Primary event			
Local symptoms	7	9	0.5
Unusual crying	3	4	0.2
Urticaria/angioedema	31	41	2.3
Fever >40.5	6	8	0.4
Fever 38–40	5	7	0.4
Hypotonia/hyporesponsiveness	11	14	0.8
Seizures within 72 h	3	4	0.2
Guillain-Barrè within 6 weeks	1	1	0.1
Purpura	3	4	0.2
Neurological symptoms other than seizures	3	4	0.2
Anaphylaxis	1	1	0.1
Gastrointestinal symptoms	1	1	0.1
hypothermia	1	1	0.1
Concomitant event			
None	62	82	4.5
Local symptoms	2	3	0.1
Unusual crying	1	1	0.1
Urticaria/angioedema	1	1	0.1
Fever >40.5	2	3	0.1
Fever 38–40	4	5	0.3
Hypotonia/hyporesponsiveness	1	1	0.1
Seizures within 72 h	2	3	0.1
Gastrointestinal symptoms	1	1	0.1
VAEs characteristics			
Severity grade 1	13		17
Severity grade 2	54		71
Severity grade 3	9		12
Time interval Mean, ±SD	26 h		72 h
Time interval Median, range	6 h		10 min to 480 h
VAE duration Mean, ±SD	82 h		189 h
VAE duration Median, range	48 h		30 min to 24 h
N. hospitalization	19		25

	N reported events	% on reported events[a]	% on observed patients[b]
N. vaccinated that reported sequelae	0		-
N. positive familiar history for VAEs	16		21

[a]Percentage of events with respect to the number of patients with VAE (n. 76).
[b]Percentage of events with respect to the observed at-risk patients (n. 1367).

Table 1. List of characteristics and types of VAEs.

and referred VAE was 26 ± 72 h. The mean duration of referred VAE was 82 ± 189 h. The longest referred VAEs were obviously Guillain-Barrè syndrome, which lasted 60 days. Nineteen out of 76 patients (25%) had been hospitalized after the previous VAE. No patient reported permanent sequela after the referred VAE (**Table 1**).

Correlation between specific vaccine(s) and kind of VAE: We found that the coadministration of hexavalent and PCV13 is the most commonly reported VAE (47 patients, 62.7%), followed by hexavalent alone (7 patients, 9%), MMR (5 patients, 6.7%), and DTaP (4 patients, 5%) (**Table 2**).

Type of reaction caused by specific vaccine(s): Coadministration of hexavalent and PCV 13 was most commonly associated with urticaria/angioedema (21 patients) and hypotonia/hyporesponsiveness (8 patients). Administration of hexavalent alone was associated with various kinds of VAE (hypotonia/hyporesponsiveness, local symptoms, urticaria/angioedema, fever >40.5 grades, anaphylaxis, and fever 38–40 grades). MMR administration was associated with urticaria/angioedema, fever 38–40 grades, fever >40.5 grades, and Guillain-Barrè syndrome. DTaP administration was followed by local symptoms in 2 patients, and irritability or urticaria/angioedema in 1 patient each (**Table 2**).

Type of reaction	Hexavalen	DTaP/ IPV	Hex+PCV	PCV13	MenB	MMR	Var	MeC cayw	Flu	HPV	tot
Local symptoms	1	2	4	1	1	-	-	-	-	-	**9**
Unusual crying	-	-	4	-	-	-	-	-	-	-	**4**
Urticaria/ angioedema	1	1	21	-	2	3	1	3	-	-	**32**
Fever >4.5	1	-	6	-	-	-	-	-	1	-	**8**
Fever	3	-	5	-	-	1	-	-	-	-	**9**
Hypotonia/ hyporesponsiveness	1	-	9	-	-	1	-	-	-	1	**12**
Seizures within 72 h	-	-	4	-	-	-	-	-	1	-	**5**
Guillain-Barré within 6 weeks	-	-	-	-	-	1	-	-	-	-	**1**

Type of reaction	Hexavalen	DTaP/ IPV	Hex+PCV	PCV13	MenB	MMR	Var	MeC cayw	Flu	HPV	tot
Purpura	-	-	1	1	-	-	-	1	-	-	**3**
Irritability	-	1	2	-	-	-	-	-	-	-	**3**
Anaphylaxis	1	-	-	-	-	-	-	-	-	-	**1**
Gastrointestinal symptoms	-	-	2	-	-	-	-	-	-	-	**2**
Hypothermia	-	-	1	-	-	-	-	-	-	-	**1**
Total events by vaccine type	**8**	**4**	**59**	**2**	**3**	**6**	**1**	**4**	**2**	**1**	**90**
Percentage of events by type	**8.9**	**4.4**	**65.5**	**2.2**	**3.3**	**6.7**	**1.1**	**4.4**	**2.2**	**1.1**	**%**

Table 2. Vaccine adverse events by the type of vaccine.

3.2. Revaccination in Bambino Gesù Children Hospital

All patients that came to our unit with a history of VAE were evaluated for eligibility to continue the vaccination schedule or to be revaccinated with further dose of the same vaccine. Out of the total number of 76 patients, 31 (41%) patients described a VAE of suspected allergic origin (i.e., urticaria/angioedema, anaphylaxis). Our approach to revaccination in patients that referred VAEs of suspected allergic nature is summarized in **Table 3**. All of these 31 patients underwent a skin prick test before revaccination with the same or a different vaccine: all skin tests resulted negative. All patients within our sample were further vaccinated one or more times. None experienced adverse events again.

Type of VAE	N° VAEs (%)	Vaccine causing the referred VAE	N°	Same vaccine	Subunit of the same vaccine	Different type of vaccine	Same vaccine or subunit + different vaccine	Recurrent VAE
Urticaria/ angioedema	32 (42%)	Hexavalent + PCV13	21	4	6	5	6	None
		DTaP	1	0	0	1	0	None
		Hexavalent	1	0	0	1	0	None
		MenB	2	2	0	0	0	None
		MenC	2	0	0	0	2	None
		MMR	3	0	0	3	0	None
		Varicella	1	0	1	0	0	None
		Men ACWY + B	1	0	0	0	0	None
Anaphylaxis	1 (1%)	Hexavalent	1	0	0	1	0	None

Table 3. Immunization of allergic patients with a previous VAE.

4. Discussion

In this report, we describe our experience with patients having a history of VAE who come to medical attention for vaccination counseling. In agreement with literature data, our findings show that VAEs are not common and that severe reactions are particularly rare [27]. Our data also demonstrate that VAEs are not recurring events, in general. This information should be shared with parents and patients, since they are often worried that VAE might reappear after subsequent vaccination events. Indeed, this is the most common reason leading to revaccination refusal [9] and noncompletion of vaccination schedules [28].

The only specific risk of repeated VAEs regards those of allergic nature, in particular VAEs that can be interpreted as acute allergic reactions (i.e., IgE-mediated). For this reason, it is important to perform accurate anamnesis and SPT in patients with referred VAEs of suspected allergic nature, using particular caution with patients who exhibit positive SPT (none in our sample). In 2010, Fritsche et al. have accurately described a diagnostic and therapeutic approach toward children with suspected vaccine allergy, highlighting the important role of STP and exposing the desensitization criteria to be employed for revaccination [29]. Based on our experience, when first reactions occur at a very young age and with more than one vaccine, revaccinations are best approached "step by step," with no more than one vaccine per visit, even in cases of negative SPT.

Our analysis indicates that the most "reactogenic" vaccine is hexavalent coadministered with PCV13. This could be explained both in terms of intrinsic immunogenicity of the vaccine itself and/or with the young age of the patients [13]. It has also been demonstrated that infants who receive hexavalent plus PCV7 have almost twofold higher incidence of reactions than those who received each vaccine alone [30, 31].

VAEs were described to be severe by 12% of parents and patients in our sample, a surprisingly high number. However, we deem as important to point out that we have frequently observed that a large gap exists between parents'/patients' opinion and clinical evaluation about VAEs severity. People are often biased against and skeptical toward vaccines, and parents tend to interpret any child's symptom that appears after immunization as worrisome. This phenomenon acts as a statistical bias because probably we overestimated VAEs severity.

Two of our patients came with a history of very important VAEs. The first was a 12-year-old girl who referred a history of anaphylaxis after the third dose of hexavalent vaccine. The reaction occurred 1 h after vaccination and presented with urticaria, breathing and swallowing difficulty, and vomiting. The patient was brought to an emergency department where she was treated with epinephrine, fluids, and steroids. She was discharged after 3 days of hospitalization, in good health conditions. She and her parents denied any history of allergy. After this episode, her vaccine calendar was interrupted. In our vaccine unit, she was re-vaccinated with MMR, after STP with the vaccine had resulted to be negative. Although she did not experience any VAE, she will be re-evaluated to decide whether she can undergo re-vaccination with DTaP. The second patient who referred to our center with a history of serious VAE was a 7-year-old girl with a previous history of Guillain-Barrè syndrome, which had occurred after the administration of the second dose of MMR. The syndrome appeared 3 weeks after vaccination with leg weakness that led to walking impossibility within a few hours. She was admitted to the neurology department of our hospital, where she was promptly diagnosed and received immunoglobulin treatment. She was discharged after a period of 20 days in good general condition and did not experience any sequela nor relapse of the syndrome. After this episode, she did not receive any other vaccine. In our unit, she was re-vaccinated following the routinary vaccination calendar and did not experience any further VAE.

Recent reports discuss the classification of VAEs and clarify the correct interpretation of the linkage between an adverse event and previous vaccination [11]; some authors propose algorithms to assess the linkage between VAE and vaccine [32]. According to those indications, a VAE is defined to be caused by the immunization if it is linked to a vaccine product-related reaction, a vaccine quality defect-related reaction, an immunization error-related reaction, and an immunization anxiety-related reaction. Other VAEs are defined as indeterminately related with the immunization, inconsistently related with the immunization and unclassifiable. WHO published a causality assessment manual in which it is possible to follow a causality assessment checklist to clarify the linkage between events and immunizations [10]. Indian guidelines classify VAEs in five broad categories: programmatic error, vaccine reaction, injection reactions, coincidental, and unknown [33]. It is particularly important to distinguish between VAEs that are actually related to the vaccination (i.e., caused by the vaccination, indeterminately related to it, programmatic error, vaccine reaction, or injection reaction) and others, because the second are not reproducible and do not represent a contraindication to re-vaccination. Clinicians should be familiar with these differences and encourage parents and patients to re-vaccination when they refer VAE of the coincidental type. Following those schemes, patients in our sample reported VAEs that could be interpreted as being related to the vaccination, such as allergic and local reactions, as well as VAEs with indeterminate relation with the vaccination, such as fever and unusual crying. It must be empathized that the first group comprises VAEs that are potentially reproducible and patients who should always be studied before re-vaccination (by anamnesis, physical findings, and SPT). Conversely, the second group includes VAEs that are rarely reproduced and patients that can almost always be safely re-vaccinated. As far as our two cases of severe VAE are concerned, anaphylaxis was related to vaccination and Guillain-Barrè syndrome had an indeterminate relation with it. Both patients were re-vaccinated, but we considered it to be important to make SPT before re-vaccination of the first patient and have not administered the causative vaccine of anaphylaxis yet. Notably, both patients had interrupted their vaccine calendar before coming to our attention, but re-vaccination resulted to be safe and neither of them experienced any complication.

5. Conclusion

In conclusion, we wish to empathize the concept that a history of VAE does not necessarily represent a contraindication to re-vaccination, as well as encourage clinicians to take advantage of algorithms for VAEs assessment to evaluate the risk of reproducibility. It should be underlined that no classification provides certain proof in favor or against the existence of an association between an event and an immunization. Nevertheless, they provide valuable assistance to clinicians in the determination of the level of likelihood of specific associations.

To maintain public confidence in vaccines, it is important that advanced immunization programs include pre- and postvaccination counseling for subjects at risk [34, 35].

In Italy, VAEs surveillance is mandatory and spontaneous reports of Adverse Events Following Immunization (AEFI) are collected by the National Network of Pharmaco-vigilance, which includes the Italian Medicine Agency, the 20 regions and autonomous provinces of Trento and Bolzano, 204 local health units, 112 hospitals, 38 research institutes, and 561 pharmaceutical industries [36]. Every clinician and vaccine service should contribute to this surveillance and have access to all required data for accurate counseling to parents and patients, and to reassure them about the safety and importance of vaccines. In this era of widespread skepticism about vaccines, easily accessible as well as rigorous counseling is required more than ever.

Acknowledgements

We thank all our colleagues and nurses in particular A. Serpi, L. Varanese, and R. Montanaro who provided insight and expertise that greatly assisted this research.

Glossary

VAE: any medical incident that takes place after immunization and is believed to be caused by the immunization itself. It is considered any unfavorable or unintended sign, and any abnormal laboratory finding, symptom, or disease

Causality assessment: linkage between a medical incident and a vaccine. Many authors have proposed causality assessment schemes that can be applied to help clinicians distinguish between events whose association with the vaccination is consistent, indeterminate, or inconsistent

Event caused by the immunization: an event that is attributable to a vaccine product-related reaction, a vaccine quality defect-related reaction, an immunization error-related reaction, and an immunization anxiety-related reaction

Coincidental adverse event: medical event that occurs after immunization but it is not caused by immunization itself, and would have occurred independently from the vaccination. In the case of coincidental adverse events, the relation between event and vaccine is only temporally

Temporal association: time interval between the vaccination and the adverse event. Temporal association is independent from causality and events that are temporally associated with vaccines that may or may not be caused by the vaccines

Serious VAE: any VAE that causes a potential risk to the life/health of the recipient, that leads to hospitalization, and that causes disability/incapacity/congenital anomaly or birth defect.

Minor VAE: an event that is not serious and has no potential risk to the health of the recipient of the vaccine

Reproducibility risk: risk that a VAE could reappear after another dose of the same/of another vaccine. The reproducibility risk is mostly significant for VAEs of allergic nature.

Vaccine pharmaco-vigilance: the science of detection, assessment, understanding, and communication of VAEs and other vaccine-related issues

Immunization anxiety-related reaction: an event that arises from anxiety about immunization

Immunization error-related reaction: an event that is caused by an inappropriate vaccine handling, prescribing, or administration

Vaccine product-related reaction: an event that is attributable to one or more properties of the vaccine product, whether the active component or one of the other components of the vaccine (adjuvants, preservatives, stabilizers)

Vaccine quality defect-related reaction: an event that is attributable to one or more quality defects of the vaccine product, including defects of the administration devices

Author details

Guido Castelli Gattinara*, Elena Bellelli, Donatella F. Angelone, Veronica Santilli and Luciana Nicolosi

*Address all correspondence to: guido.castelli@opbg.net

Vaccination Center, Pediatric University-Hospital Department, Bambino Gesù Pediatric Hospital, IRCCS, Rome, Italy

References

[1] World Health Organization. AEFI Investigation. Available from: http://www.who.int/vaccine_safety/publications/AEFI_Investigation_Aide_Memoire.pdf

[2] World Health Organization. Surveillance of Adverse Events Following Immunization, Field Guide for Managers of Immunization Programs. Geneva: World Health Organization; 1997

[3] Definitions and Applications Terms on Pharmacovigilance. Report of CIOMS/WHO Working Group on Vaccine Pharmacovigilance. WHO Oct 2012; http://www.who.int/vaccine_safety/initiative/tools/CIOMS_report_WG_vaccine.pdf

[4] Introduction to VAERS, CDC, FDA. https://www.cdc.gov/vaccinesafety/ensuringsafety/monitoring/vaers

[5] Weekly epidemiological record. Releve epidemiologicque hebdomadaire. WHO. 2016; **3**(91):21-32

[6] MacDonalds NE, Finlay JC. Working with vaccine hesitant parents. Paediatrics and Child Health. 2013;**18**(5):265-267

[7] Federman R. Understanding vaccines: A public imperative. Yale Journal of Biology and Medicine. 2014;**87**(4):417-422

[8] Capanna A, Gervasi G, Ciabattini M, et al. Effects of mass media on influenza vaccine coverage in the season 2014/2015: A regional survey in Lazio, Italy. Journal of Preventive Medicine and Hygiene (JPMH). 2015;**56**(2):E72-E76

[9] Chitkara AJ, Thacker N, Vashishtha MN, et al. Adverse Event Following Immunization (AEFI) Surveillance in India: Position Paper of Indian Academy of Pediatrics. Indian Pediatrics. 2015;**50**:739-741

[10] WHO/HIS/EMP/QSS. Causality Assessment of an Adverse Event Following Immunization (AEFI). User Manual for the Revised WHO Classification. WHO; 2013. www.who.int/vaccine_safety/publications/aevi_manual.pdf

[11] Gold MS, Balakrishnan MR, Amarasinghe A, et al. An approach to death as an adverse event following immunization. Vaccine. 2016;**34**:212-217

[12] Ruggeberg JU, Gold MS, Bayas J-M, et al. Anaphylaxis: Case definition and guidelines for data collection, analysis, and presentation of immunization safety data. Vaccine. 2007;**25**(31):5675-5684

[13] Nicolosi L, Vittucci A, Mancini R, et al. Vaccine risk assessment in children with a referred reaction to a previous vaccine dose: 2009-2011 retrospective report at the Bambino Gesu' children hospital, Rome, Italy. Italian Journal of Pediatrics. 2014;**40**(31):1-8

[14] Echeverría-Zudaire LA, Ortigosa del Castillo L, Alonso Lebrero E, et al. Consensus document on the approach to children with allergic reactions after vaccination or allergy to vaccine components. Allergologia et Immunopathologia (Madrid). 2015;**43**(3):304-325

[15] National Health and Medical Research Council. The Australian Immunisation Handbook. 6th ed. Canberra: AGPS; 1997

[16] Burgess M, McIntyre P, Heath T. Rethinking the contraindications to vaccination. Medical Journal. 1998;**168**:476-477

[17] Franceschini F, Bottau P, Caimmi S, et al. Vaccination in children allergic to non active vaccine components. Clinical and Translational Medicine. 2015;**14**(4):1-8

[18] Gold M. Hypotonic-hyporesponsive episodes following pertussis vaccination. A cause of concern?. Drug Safety. 2002;**25**(2):85-90

[19] Gold R, Scheifele D, Halperin S, et al. Hypotonic-hyporesponsive episodes in children hospitalized at 10 Canadian Pediatric Tertiary-Care Centres, 1991-1994. Canada Communicable Disease Report. 1997;**23**(10):73-76

[20] Bitnun A, Shannon P, Durward A, et al. Measles inclusion-body encephalitis caused by the vaccine strain of measles virus. Clinical Infectious Diseases. 1999;**29**(4):855-861

[21] Rennels MB, Deloria MA, Pichichero ME, et al. Extensive swelling after booster doses of acellular pertussis–tetanus–diphtheria vaccines. Pediatrics. 2000;**105**(e12):1-6

[22] Pichichero ME, Edwards KM, Anderson EL, et al. Safety and immunogenicity of six acellular pertussis vaccines and one whole-cell pertussis vaccine given as a fifth dose in four to six year old children. Pediatrics. 2000;**105**(1):1-8

[23] Marshall H, Nolan T, Roberton D, et al. A comparison of booster immunisation with a combination DTPa-IPV vaccine or DTPa plus IPV in separate injections when co-administered with MMR, at age 4-6 years. Vaccine. 2006;**24**:6120-6128

[24] Jacquet JM, Bégué P, Grimprel E, et al. Safety and immunogenicity of a combined DTPa-IPV vaccine administered as a booster from 4 years of age: A review. Vaccine. 2006;**24**(13):2440-2448

[25] Gold MS, Noonan S, Osbourn M, et al. Local reactions after fourth-dose of acellular pertussis vaccine in South Australia. Medical Journal of Australia. 2003;**179**(4):191-194

[26] Taddio A, McMurtry CM, Shah V, et al. Reducing pain during vaccine injections: Clinical practice guideline. Canadian Medical Association Journal. 2015;**187**(13):975-982

[27] American Academy of Pediatrics: Active Immunization. In: Pickering LK, Baker CJ, Long SS, McMillan JA, editors. Red Book 2006 Report of the Committee on Infectious Diseases. 27th ed. Elk Grove Village, IL: American Academy of Pediatrics; 2006. pp. 446-448

[28] Gold M, Goodwin H, Botham S, et al. Re-vaccination of 421 children with a past history of adverse vaccine reaction in a special immunization service. Archives of Disease in Childhood. 2000;**83**:128-131

[29] Fritsche FP, Helbling A, Ballmer-Weber BK. Vaccine hypersensitivity, update and overview. Swiss Medical Weekly. 2010;**140**(17-18):238-246

[30] Knuf M, Habermehl P, Cimino C, et al. Immunogenicity, reactogenicity and safety of a 7-valent pneumococcal conjugate vaccine [PCV7) concurrently administered with a DTPa-HBV-IPV/Hib combination vaccine in healthy infants. Vaccine. 2006;**24**:4727-4736

[31] Olivier C, Belohradsky BH, Stojanov S, et al. Immunogenicity, reactogenicity, and safety of a seven-valent pneumococcal conjugate vaccine (PCV7) concurrently administered with a fully liquid DTPa-IPV-HBV-Hib combination vaccine in healthy infants. Vaccine. 2008;**26**:3142-3152

[32] Halsey NA, Edwards KM, Dekker CL, et al. Algorithm to assess causality after an individual adverse event following immunizations. Vaccine. 2012;**30**:5792-5798

[33] Government of India. Adverse Events Following Immunization: Surveillance and Response Operational Guidelines. New Delhi: Ministry of Health and Family Welfare, Government of India; 2010

[34] Mullooly JP, Thompson RS, Bohlke K, et al. Risk of anaphylaxis after vaccination of children and adolescents. Vaccine Safety Datalink Team, Pediatrics. 2003;**112**(4):815-820

[35] Advisory Committee on Immunization Practices (ACIP): General Recommendations on Immunization. MMWR Recommendations and Reports. National Center for Immunization and Respiratory Diseases; 2011;Vol. **60**. N2

[36] Alicino C, Merlano C, Zampettini S, et al. Routine surveillance of adverse events following immunization as important tool to monitor vaccine safety. Human Vaccines & Immunotherapeutics. 2015;**11**(1):91-94